FIRST EDITION

D1216939

INFORMATION TECHNOLOGY IN HEALTHCARE

WHAT PROFESSIONALS NEED TO KNOW

By Min Wu

University of Wisconsin - Milwaukee

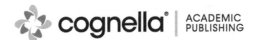
cognella® | ACADEMIC PUBLISHING

Bassim Hamadeh, CEO and Publisher

Kassie Graves, Director of Acquisitions

Jamie Giganti, Senior Managing Editor

Jess Estrella, Senior Graphic Designer

Mark Combes, Senior Field Acquisitions Editor

Sean Adams, Project Editor

Luiz Ferreira, Senior Licensing Specialist

Allie Kiekhofer, Associate Editor

Kevin Fontimayor, Interior Designer

Cover image copyright © iStockphoto LP/xijian.

Printed in the United States of America

ISBN: 978-1-63487-634-6 (pbk) / 978-1-63487-635-3 (br)

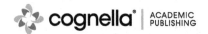

Contents

01

Introduction to Biomedical Informatics

What Is Biomedical Informatics?

A short answer to this question is "the application of Information Technology (IT) to health care." There are many definitions of this new interdisciplinary field. Some technology-oriented definitions focus on the IT applications, such as electronic medical records and hospital-information systems. Some definitions describe various roles biomedical informatics can play within health care, such as optimizing the use of health information. The purpose of this book is to provide a conceptual introduction to the field of biomedical informatics. A conceptually oriented definition has been proposed as follows: "Medical informatics is the discipline concerned with the systematic processing of data, information, and knowledge in medicine and health care" [1]. Informatics is the methodology, or way of approaching problems, while the areas of interest are medicine and health care.

Subfields in Biomedical Informatics [2]

Based on the level of research targets, we use more narrow terms for specific areas of study in biomedical informatics. When research targets are molecular and cellular processes, we call it bioinformatics or genomics. Imaging informatics has a focus on imaging tissues and organs. Clinical informatics generally refers to informatics applied in clinical settings, including nursing (nursing informatics), dentistry (dental informatics), pathology

1

(pathology informatics) and other clinical specialties. The focus of consumer health informatics is informatics from the consumer point of view. When the research targets are populations, it is public health informatics. It is the application of informatics in areas of public health, including surveillance, reporting, and health promotion. The more general term health informatics refers to both clinical informatics and public health informatics.

What Is Data?

In this book, the definition of data is narrowed and different from the broad "data" concept we use every day. For example, data could be "Edwin," "blood pressure," "140," and "90." Those elements are data and can be stored in a computer. An individual data item is meaningless in itself. A number, such as "140," can be anything if we do not know what it refers to.

What Is Information?

The information is meaningful sentences in human languages. Data can be used to form meaningful propositions or information, such as "Edwin's blood pressure is 140 over 90." Every day, we are creating and sharing information. Information is what we want. Information retrieval is the key skill we should have.

Data Versus Information

Information in human languages is what we really care about. For example, medical records are critical for physicians to provide patient care and must include a patient's vital information, such as blood pressure. A computer is designed to manage information and help our limited human memory. The relationship among data, information, and computer is shown in Figure 1.1.

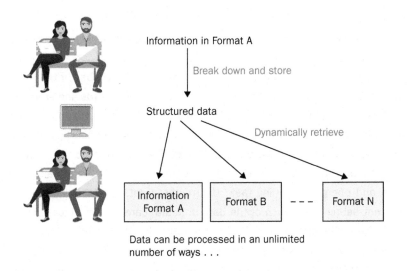

Information in Format A

Break down and store

Structured data

Dynamically retrieve

| Information Format A | Format B | – – – | Format N |

Data can be processed in an unlimited number of ways . . .

Figure 1.1. Data, Information, and Computer

We can break down a piece of information in Format A (such as, "Melvin's blood pressure is 140 over 90.") into individual data elements (such as "Melvin," "140," "90," etc). A computer can store those data elements for us. If the data is well organized in a computer, and it can be searched, we refer to the data as "structured data." The structured data elements can be dynamically retrieved and processed in unlimited ways. For example, we are able to provide different views of medical records, such as time-oriented, location-oriented, and problem-oriented. We also can present the information visually, using charts and graphs. In order to optimize use of the information, we need to break down old information first, store structured data in the computer, and retrieve and dynamically construct new information for different uses.

Information Explosion and Big Data

In our age, information explosion leads to information overload or too much information. Some information is kept in paper-based records and stored in folders in cabinets (see Figure 1.2). More information is created and stored in digital formats, such as emails. In this era of social media, millions of messages, photos, and posts are published every second. To find specific information on a subject from both paper-based records and emails is a time and energy-consuming task. Unstructured data is not well-organized and not searchable. Much of the data in health care is unstructured, such as electronic health-records notes, clinical trial research, medical images, and medical sensor streams. The challenge is that the speed of producing unstructured data is so fast, and the data cannot be processed into a structured format in a timely fashion. More and more information or unstructured data is filed in storage and archive systems. After the unstructured data goes to the archives, most likely, it will be forgotten and never will be used in the future. This is the "Big Data" issue. The increasing Big Data volume, velocity, and variety require novel technologies to process the data and analyze useful information.

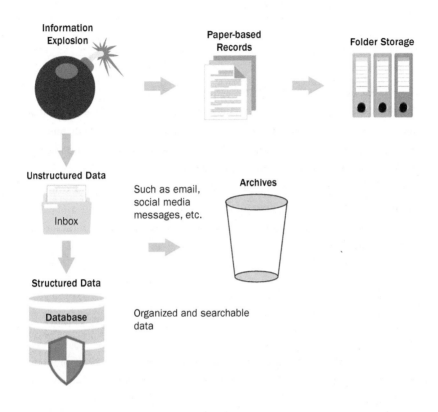

Figure 1.2. Information Explosion and Big Data

Data volume is growing exponentially in the biomedical informatics fields. The new generation of sequencing technologies is capable of producing billions of DNA sequences per day at a relatively low cost, and the growth of this technology is expected to increase. Many scientists predict that personalized medicine based on a patient's whole genome sequencing will soon become affordable. On the clinical side, a tremendous volume of patient data has been collected and stored in an electronic format. Public health researchers could take advantage of the social media data to discover new patterns among population groups.

What Is Knowledge?

Knowledge can be facts derived through the interpretation of data. Normally, documented knowledge refers to study results in the literature. A clinical guideline is an example of medical knowledge, such as "Hypertension: blood pressure > 140/90." Hypertension is the condition diagnosed when a patient's blood pressure reading is higher than normal. The American Heart Association has long considered blood pressure less than 140 over 90 normal for adults. Another source of knowledge is the expert in a specific domain who has skills acquired through experience or the understanding of a subject.

Information, Database and Knowledge Base

The purpose of biomedical informatics training programs is to produce information architects who know where information comes from and where information will go to. We really care about patients' health information and study workflows in clinics. For example, in clinics, the nurse starts collecting information, such as chief complaints, and measures patients' vital signs, such as body temperature and blood pressure. To optimize collecting and retrieving information, we design computer applications with user-friendly interfaces to help healthcare providers.

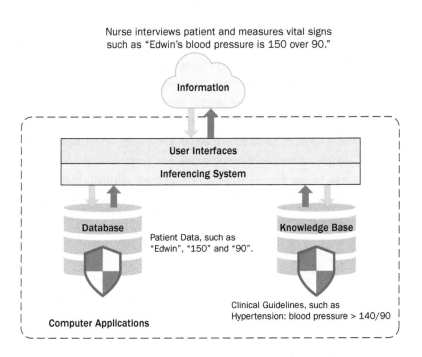

Nurse interviews patient and measures vital signs such as "Edwin's blood pressure is 150 over 90."

Information

User Interfaces

Inferencing System

Database

Patient Data, such as "Edwin", "150" and "90".

Knowledge Base

Clinical Guidelines, such as Hypertension: blood pressure > 140/90

Computer Applications

Figure 1.3. Information, Database and Knowledge Base

On the back end (server side) of computer applications, we create databases to organize data. Patients' structured data is stored in the database, such as "Edwin," "150," and "90." In this book, several chapters will focus on database-related concepts and skills, starting from data acquisition to logical and physical designs of a new database. In logical design, we will study basic concepts of data models. We also learn skills to develop a new relational data model using Entity Relationship (ER) diagrams and skills of Normalizations to improve previous data model design. In physical design, we will introduce the concepts of indexes and performance tuning in Database Management System (DBMS).

On the server side of computer applications, we also develop a knowledge base to systematically organize medical knowledge. Making medical knowledge accessible and interpretable electronically is still a challenging task. It includes both knowledge acquisition, such as machine learning, and knowledge engineering. In addition, we need to design specific software for knowledge retrieval, such as "inferencing systems between patient database and medical knowledgebase." The inference engine should suggest some rules for patients whose data is delivered from a patient database and offer decisions and the reasons for these decisions (diagnosis and treatment planning). For example, clinical practice guidelines (rules) provide a rich source of up-to-date medical knowledge about best clinical practices. Hopefully, we can develop more and more clinical and genetic knowledgebase in the future. This knowledgebase will help reduce inappropriate practice variation, speed the translation of research into practice, and support quality initiatives in health care.

The Computer

The computer may be the greatest human invention ever, and it significantly changes our lives. Compared with a human, a computer has a better memory and can store and retrieve a larger amount of data. Also, computers have greater and faster computing power than the human brain, can do arithmetic calculations accurately, and do not complain about those boring repetitive computations. However, a computer is still a machine which will do only what the operator tells it to do. Computers use binary coding because the machine understands only binary codes, such as circuits open or closed, power on or off, etc. So far, computers cannot communicate with us using human languages.

Human and Computer: Natural Language Processing

An active research area in computer science is to study Natural Language Processing (NLP), which is to design and build software that will analyze, understand, and generate languages that humans use naturally.

NLP applications can extract information in text. For example, a computer can locate and structure important information in text, such as medication information in the medical records. Information retrieval is based on information extraction to access specific text in very large collections. NLP applications also can generate text by formulating natural-language sentences from structured data. For example, with an NLP application, a computer may be able to generate a small summary from a large text. In busy clinics, if a computer can generate a summary of a patient's medical records, it will be helpful for physicians to quickly review the summary before meeting the patient.

User-Interface Design

Natural language processing (NLP) could enable humans to communicate more effectively with computers. User-interface design is the most important part of human-computer interaction. For example, a user-friendly computer interface will support natural language searches, such as, "What could cause high blood pressure?" Based on the research of biomedical informatics, we could design the computer application to replace everyday words ("high blood pressure") with specific medical terms ("hypertension") to increase matches in medical literature.

Speech (Voice) Recognition in Health care

Speech (Voice) Recognition is a part of natural language processing. Voice recognition can be applied to health care. For example, in a quiet room in a hospital, a radiologist can record his/her interpretations of medical images. Because there are limited vocabularies in radiology diagnosis reports, we have encouraging results using voice recognition technology to communicate between radiologists and computers. However, in busy clinics with a lot of noise, it will be a huge challenge for computers to understand human voices.

Computer Application

A computer application includes three components: input, process, and output (see Figure 1.4). The computer runs a process that gets inputs related to a task and outputs data which represents the result of executing the task.

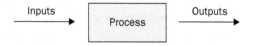

Figure 1.4. Computer Application

Abstract

In order to develop a computer application, we need to abstract the real-world task into application programming interfaces (APIs), such as input, process, and output. For example, we can abstract TV for end users into "Power on/off," "Volume up/down," or "Channel +/-." For a complex large task, we simply divide it into several small tasks. In Figure 1.5, multiple layers of APIs are developed. The output of the first API will become the input of the second API.

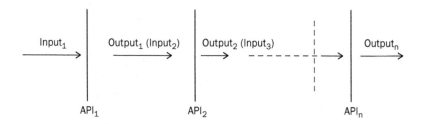

Figure 1.5. Application Program Interfaces (APIs)

To abstract the behaviors of a customer in a bank, we can successfully design computer applications to deposit, borrow, or withdraw money. In clinical medicine, we must be prepared to analyze complex behaviors that humans display and to describe patients as completely as possible. In general, medical information in the high-level description tends to be soft or fuzzy. This is why it will be a challenging task to abstract health-related situations and develop computer applications in health care. Complete implementation of artificial intelligence in medicine is probably a long way off. Most likely, these days we are working on simple computer-aided decision-support components.

A Case Study: Body Mass Index (BMI)

One of widely used health indicators is Body Mass Index (BMI). It has four categories as follows:

- Underweight = < 18.5
- Normal weight = 18.5-24.9
- Overweight   = 25-29.9
- Obesity = BMI of 30 or greater

In this case study, we will design a computer application to calculate BMI which includes three components: Input, process and output.

Input:
1. Given that height is 5' 09" and weight is 150 pounds.
2. Convert to standard units:
    $H = (5 + 9/12) \text{ foot} * 0.3048 \text{m/foot} = 1.75 \text{ (m)}$
    $W = 150 \text{ Pound} * 0.454 \text{ kg/pound} = 68.1 \text{ (kg)}$

Process:

3. Calculate BMI using a given equation:
    $BMI = Weight / (Height * Height) = 68.1/(1.75*1.75) = 22$

Outputs:
4. Compare with BMI Categories.

The patient's weight is with BMI at 22.

Organization of the Text

When information technology is referenced, the first thing that comes to mind is probably databases and the Internet. When healthcare information technology is mentioned, the first thing that comes to mind is electronic medical records. In addition to these topics, it will be helpful for you to have an overall understanding of software engineering and to know something about how software is developed. In the five sections or parts of this book, we will cover four components of medical informatics: databases (Part I and Part III), electronic medical records (Part II), the network (Part IV), and software engineering (Part V).

References

Hasman, A., R. Haux, and A. Albert. "A Systematic View on Medical Informatics," *Comput Methods Programs Biomed 51* (Nov. 1996). 131-9.

Hersh, W. "A Stimulus to Define Informatics and Health Information Technology," *BMC Medical Informatics and Decision Making* 9 (2009), 24.

Credits

1.1a   Man and woman using laptop: Copyright © Depositphotos/royalty.

1.1b   Office icons: Copyright © Depositphotos/vectorikart.

1.2a   Security Flat Colored Icons 4: Copyright © Depositphotos/educester.

1.2b   Office icons: Copyright © Depositphotos/vectorikart.

1.2c   Documents: Copyright © Depositphotos/fad82.

1.2d   Color business collection: Copyright © Depositphotos/4zeva.

1.3a   Security Flat Colored Icons 4: Copyright © Depositphotos/educester.

Data Model and Design Process

What Is a Database (DB)?

A database is an organized collection of data [1]. Why we need to study databases? The short answer is that data is everywhere. Datasets are increasing in diversity and volume. For example, data is growing in digital libraries. The Human Genome Project has new datasets about human gene sequences. Wearable technology, such as Google Watch, generates data about movement, heart rate, etc. every day.

What Is a Database Management System (DBMS)?

A database management system (DBMS) is a software program used to create, maintain, modify, and manipulate a database. Currently, major DBMS Vendors are Oracle, IBM (DB2), Microsoft (Access, SQL Server) and so on. These systems must be purchased, installed and set up for particular applications.

What Is a Database Application?

A database application is a collection of data and programs that allow the manipulation of these data (see Figure 2.1). For example, the banking system is a database application to handle banking data, such as information on accounts, customers, balances, current interest rates, transaction histories, etc. The Amazon website (Amazon.com) relies heavily on databases and is a web-based database application. Stock-monitoring systems are real-time "active" databases.

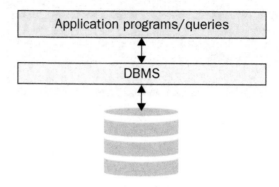

Figure 2.1. Database Application

Who Works With Databases?

Every day we work with databases. As end users of database, we query databases through application-user interfaces, such as Google search. Database designers are people who design database "schema" to model aspects of the real world. Database-application developers are people who build applications that interface with databases. Database administrators will load, back up, restore data and fine-tune databases for performances. DBMS vendors are software companies who develop the DBMS or specialized data-management software and implement new techniques for query processing and optimization inside DBMS.

What Is a Data Model?

Models are a cornerstone of design. For example, engineers build a model of car to work out any details before putting it into production. We will develop models to explore ideas and improve the understanding of the database design. Models help communicate the concepts in people's minds. The purposes are to communicate, categorize, describe, specify, investigate, evolve, analyze, and imitate.

Four Types of Data Models

To abstract the real world, there are four basic data models as follows:

Hierarchical Data Model: It has a tree of sets of records (see Figure 2.2). The tree starts from the root node. Each child node has only one parent node, whereas each parent node can have one or more child nodes. In order to retrieve data from this model, the whole tree needs to be traversed starting from the root node.

Figure 2.2. Hierarchical Data Model

Network Data Model: Any record in this model could be a parent/child relationship or a peer-level relationship (See Figure 2.3), so multiple relationships could exist between all kinds of records. Anything can point to anything. Just like the Web, it is impossible to predict or control these relationships between websites and URLs because it is so easy to set links between things.

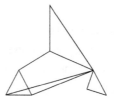

Figure 2.3. Network Data Model

Relational Data Model: This model uses a simple data structure: the table (see Figure 2.4). It is the only data structure in this model. A table has a specified number of columns but can have any number of rows.

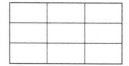

Figure 2.4. Relational Data Model

Object-oriented Data Model: This model encapsulates data and programs into an object (see Figure 2.5). Any real-world entity is uniformly modeled as an object. Every object has the set of values for the attributes of the object and the set of methods/functions which operate on the attributes of the object.

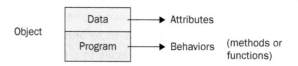

Figure 2.5. Object-oriented Data Model

What Is a "Software Crisis"?

"Software crisis" in the software-engineering field is a term used to describe the difficulty of writing useful and efficient computer programs in the required time. Eighty to ninety percent of systems do not meet their performance goals. About eighty percent are delivered late and over budget. Around forty percent of developments fail or are abandoned. Less than forty percent of systems fully address training and skills requirements. Less than twenty-five percent of systems properly integrate business and technology objectives. Just ten to twenty percent of systems meet all their success criteria. What happened? Major reasons are the lack of complete requirement specifications, the lack of an appropriate development methodology, and poor decomposition of design into manageable components.

The Database Design Process

In order to successfully develop a database, we need to have an appropriated development methodology. In another words, we should design a new database systematically. Figure 2.6 illustrates one of the process models to develop a database. [1]

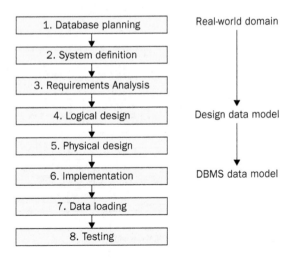

Figure 2.6. Database-design Processes

Database Planning: In the first phase, we need to conduct interviews with main users in the real-world domain to create mission statements and objectives. Begin with the end result in mind. The mission statement defines the major aims of the database application. Here is an example of a mission statement: "The purpose of the NLM educational database application in breast imaging at UNC is to maintain the data that we generate, to support the educational tools for radiologists who interpret mammograms, and to facilitate cooperation and sharing of information between universities." Each mission objective identifies a particular task that the database must support. Here is a further example of mission objectives:

- To perform searches on mammogram cases, users, and tests.
- To create mammogram test sets and ROC data analysis.
- To track the status of breast images, test items, and users.
- To report on mammography cases, tests, and users; to provide evaluation of users' performance in interpreting mammography; to provide user feedback from the online survey.

System Definition: System definition defines the scope and boundary of the database application, including its major user views. User view defines what is required of a database application from the perspective of a particular position (such as teacher or student). An example is shown in Figure 2.7.

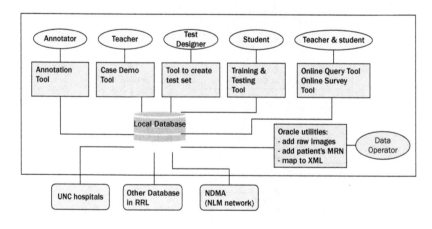

Figure 2.7. Educational Imaging System

Introduction to Healthcare Information Technology (First Edition)

Requirements for Collection and Analysis: To collect data, we can use various methods, such as user interviews, observations, and survey and document reviews. In user interviews, you need to prepare questions prior to the interview. Here are some sample interview questions:

- Who are the users for the system?
- How many users will use this system?
- Are they all in one location?
- What information would they like to get from the new database?
- What is the subject of the database?
- What kind of data is it?

Logical Design: In this phase, we need to identify the important objects that need to be represented in the database and the relationships between these objects.

Physical Design: To decide how the logical design is to be physically implemented in the target DBMS. In this course, we will learn how to create tables, relationships, forms, queries, and reports using Microsoft Access (DBMS).

Implementation: Most students in this course do not know any programming languages. We will use a graphical user interface (GUI) in Microsoft Access to implement the database design, which provides the same functionality while hiding the low-level SQL (Structured Query Language) statements.

Data Loading: We will learn how to create Access forms for data entry in this course.

Testing: Before going live, the newly developed database application should be thoroughly tested.

Reference

Hernandez, M. *Database Design for Mere Mortals: A Hands-on Guide to Relational Database Design*, 2nd edition. Boston: Addison-Wesley Longman Publishing Co., Inc. 2003.

Logical Design

What Is a Relational Database?

A database is an organized collection of data. A relational database is a collection of two-dimensional tables [1].

Here is an example of a relational database: Students in our course (see Figure 3.1). We can create several tables to store different pieces of information about students, such as a Student table and a Major table.

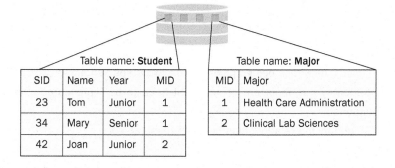

Table name: **Student**

SID	Name	Year	MID
23	Tom	Junior	1
34	Mary	Senior	1
42	Joan	Junior	2

Table name: **Major**

MID	Major
1	Health Care Administration
2	Clinical Lab Sciences

Figure 3.1. Examples of Relational Databases

There are some basic terminologies used in a relational database (see Figure 3.2). 1: A single row or tuple representing all data required for a particular student. Each row in a table should be identified by a unique identifier (primary key) which allows no duplicate rows. 2: A column or attribute containing student ID, which is also the primary key. The student ID identifies a unique student in this table. A primary key must contain a value. 3: A field can be found at the intersection of a row and a column. There can be only one value in it. 4: A field may have no value in it. This is called a null value. Mary does not have a phone number. (A null does not represent a zero or a text string of blank spaces. It's just an unknown value.)

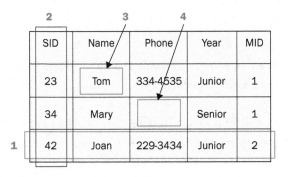

Figure 3.2. Terminology of Relational Databases

In the logical database design phase, there two steps as follows [1]:
1.   To identify the important objects that need to be represented in the database
2.   To identify the relationships between these objects.

There are key concepts in a relational database, such as entity, primary key, foreign key, etc. Let's study them one by one.

Entity: It is a thing of significance about which information needs to be known. It is an object or concept of interest and about which data is to be kept. For example, "Student" and "Major" are entities in a student database.

Attribute: Attribute is something that describes or qualifies an entity. It is a descriptive property of an entity. Attributes represent the individual elements of data that are stored and processed. For example, name, birth date and major are attributes about the Student entity (see Figure 3.3). Each of the attributes is either required or optional. It is the logical aspect. Attributes have physical aspects. For example, each attribute has a type, such as "Number," "Text," and "Date."

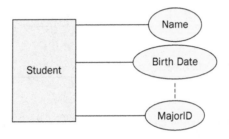

Figure 3.3. Attributes

An entity set (table) is a collection of things of the same type. Each entity set (table) has a list of attributes (columns). Each entity set (table) contains a set of records (rows). For example, "Student" and "Major" are two entities and each entity has many attributes, such as "Name," "Year," etc.

Table name: **Student**

SID	Name	Year	MID
23	Tom	Junior	1
34	Mary	Senior	1
42	Joan	Junior	2

Table name: **Major**

MID	Major
1	Health Care Administration
2	Clinical Lab Sciences

Figure 3.4. Example of Entities and Attributes

Primary Key: A primary key is a field or group of fields that uniquely identifies each record within a table. For example, student identifier (SID) can
serve as primary key for the "Student" entity (see Figure 3.5). This attribute
(SID) identifies the entity. Each SID can uniquely identify a student.

Table name: **Student**

SID	Name	Year	MID
23	Tom	Junior	1
34	Mary	Senior	1
42	Joan	Junior	2

Figure 3.5: Example of Primary Key

A combination of attributes can identify the entity. If a primary key is com-
posed of two or more fields, it is called as a composite primary key. For
example (see Figure 3.6), a combination of "Name" and "Birth Date" can
uniquely identify the student. "Name" and "Birth Date" is a composite
primary key.

Name	Birth Date	Year	MajorID
Tom	11/02/80	Junior	1
Tom	10/03/81	Senior	1
Joan	09/09/82	Junior	2

Figure 3.6. Example of Composite Primary Key

How to Identify Entities of Relational Model in a System

In order to identify entities of a system, we need to collect and analyze user-requirement data. For example, we can start with user interviews. During the user interviews, users can provide details about the samples and information about the way the organization uses data. Users are instrumental in defining preliminary field and table structures. Users help to define future information requirements. We can identify entities by analyzing the interview notes. For example, we can analyze interview notes about a lab-information system as follows:

> "A blood sample was taken by Tom on Monday using equipment at the clinical lab in the base floor of the Enderis Hall building. This blood test, conducted on that blood sample, is a new type of test, which consists of six steps. The test result is positive. The blood type of the sample is "A."

First, we can highlight important nouns as possible Entities candidates.

> "A <u>blood sample</u> was taken by <u>Tom</u> on <u>Monday</u> using <u>equipment</u> at the clinical lab in the base floor of the <u>Enderis Hall building</u>. This blood <u>test,</u> conducted on that blood sample, is a new <u>type of test</u>, which consists of six steps. The test <u>result</u> is positive. The <u>instrument</u> used in this test is a tube. The <u>blood type</u> of the sample is "A."

A list of important terms is generated:

> Blood, Sample, Tom, Monday, Equipment, Enderis Hall building, Test, Type of Test, Result, and Instrument.

We can generalize and replace some items. For example, we can use "student" to replace "Tom". "Tom" is a filed value for one record of a student.

"Blood" is a field value for one "type of sample." The list is revised as follows:

> Sample Type, Sample, Student, Date, Equipment, Location, Test, Type of Test, Result and Instrument.

After generating a preliminary table (entities) list as above, duplicate items, such as "Equipment" and "Instrument," must be resolved. Some items are attributes of an entity. For example, "Date" and "Location" describe when and where a "Test" is conducted. We will remove the attribute items from the entity list. The finalized list of entities of a general lab system is shown as follows:

- Sample
- Sample Type
- Student
- Equipment
- Test
- Type of Test
- Result

Entities vs. Attributes vs. Records

When students are identifying entities (tables) in a general lab system, they often confuse specific records (field value), attributes (column name), and entities (table names). For example, students sometimes list specific equipment names as entities, such as "Scale," "Microscope," "Test Tube," etc. Actually, "Microscope" is a record (field value) in the "Equipment" table. In addition, students may make mistakes with attributes (column names). For example, "Test Date" is an attribute to describe an entity "Test." In another words, "Test Date" (attribute) is a column name in the "Test" table (entity).

Relationships

In the logical database design phase, the first step is to identify the important objects that need to be represented in the database. The second step is to identify the relationships between these objects. The relationship

Introduction to Healthcare Information Technology (First Edition)

is used to cross reference information between tables. In general, tables can be related in one of three different ways: one-to-one, one-to-many, or many-to-many.

First, let's look at the one-to-one relationship in Figure 3.7. One table is re-lated another one and only one. For example, one car contains one engine in general. One engine is installed in one car.

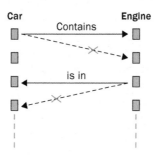

Figure 3.7. One-to-one Relationship

Second, a one-to-many relationship means that one table is related to more than one other tables. For example, one department has more than one employee (see Figure 3.8). One employee works only in one department in general.

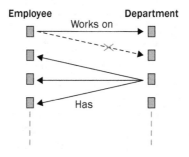

Figure 3.8. One-to-many relationship

Finally, many-to-many relationship is another type of cardinality that refers to the relationship between two tables (see Figure 3.9). For example, one student can enroll many classes. One class has many students. "Student" and "Class" have a many-to-many relationship.

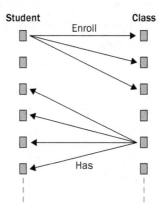

Figure 3.9. Many-to-many Relationship

Entity Relationship (ER) Diagram

A picture is worth a thousand words. We will create an entity relationship (ER) diagram to present the logical database design. The main components of ER diagrams are entities (things) and the relationships that can exist among them.

An entity (table) in an ER diagram is shown in Figure 3.10. It must include an entity (table) name and primary key (PK).

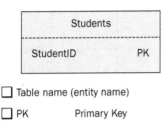

Table name (entity name)

☐ PK   Primary Key

Figure 3.10. Entity in ER

How to Implement Relationships

In order to implement relationships in relational database, we need to introduce another important concept: Foreign Key. A foreign key is a column that
defines how tables relate to each other. A foreign key refers to a primary key
in another table. We will explain foreign key concepts using entity relationship (ER) diagrams.

In order to implement a relationship, we need to create the foreign key,
a new column that defines how tables relate to each other. For example,
there is a one-to-one relationship between the "Assignment" table and
the "Grade" table. One assignment has only one grade. One grade is only
related to one assignment. We have two choices to implement a one-to-one
relationship (see Figure 3.11): (1) Creating a new column, "R_AssignID,"
as a foreign key in the "Grade" table, which refers to a primary key in
the "Assignment" table; or (2) Creating a new column, "R_GradeID," as a
foreign key in the "Assignment" table, which refers to a primary key in the
"Grade" table.

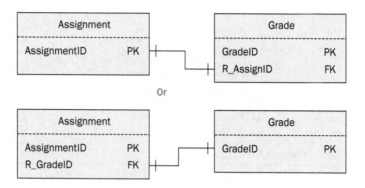

Figure 3.11. One-to-one Relationship in ER

To implement a one-to-many relationship, a new column must be created as a foreign key in the "Many" side table. For example, "Department" and "Students" has a one-to-many relationship. One department has many students. One student, however, belongs to only one department. In this case, the "Many" side table is the "Student" table. A new column, "R_DeptID," is added in the "Students" table as foreign key, which refers to a primary key in the "Department" table (see Figure 3.12).

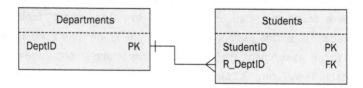

Figure 3.12. One-to-many Relationship in ER

How to Implement "Many-to-Many" Relationships

Directly implementing "many-to-many" relationships by using "foreign keys" can be difficult. For example, one class has many students, and one student may enroll in many classes. We cannot simply add a foreign key

Introduction to Healthcare Information Technology (First Edition)

to implement this relationship. The table is the only data structure in the relational database. If we cannot implement the relationship by adding new columns, we must create a new table, a linking table between the "Classes" table and the "Students" table, to solve the many-to-many relationship. It may be the most difficult part of relational-database design. In Figure 3.13, a new linking table, "Registration," forms a link between the "Classes" table and the "Students" table. One Many-to-Many relationship becomes two "one-to-many" relationships: One class has many registrations, and one student has many registrations. By adding foreign keys ("StudentID" and "ClassID") in the "Many" side table, "Registration," we successfully implement the relationships.

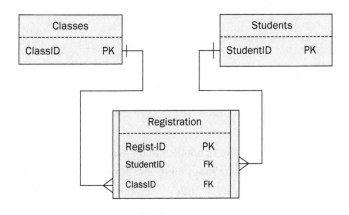

Figure 3.13 Linking Tables in ER

The above screen shot of tables ("Classes," "Students," and "Registration") with records data inside in Figure 3.14 should help you to understand the implementation of creating a new linking table to solve the "many-to-many" relationship.

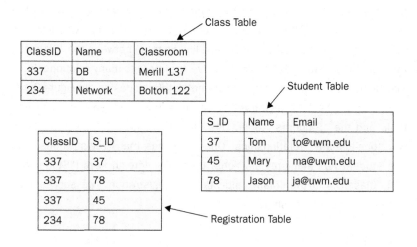

Figure 3.14 Example Tables with Records

A Case Study: Document Database

The only way to learn a skill is to practice and practice again. Here is a case scenario: In a document database, there are three entities as follows: (1) Document (with the attributes of "title," "author," etc.), (2) Document Type, such as "periodical," "drawing," etc. (3) Location, such as "UWM libraries," "bookstores," etc. Please draw an ER diagram for this system.

First, we need to draw entities ("Documents," "DocumentTypes," and "Locations") with primary keys in the ER diagram. Second, we need to find out the relationships among tables. "DocumentType" and "Documents" has a one-to-many relationship. We can add a new column, "R_TypeID," as a foreign key in the Many side table, "Documents." It is a challenge to implement the many-to-many relationship between the "Documents" table and the "Locations" table. One document has many copies in different locations. One location has many copies of one document. A new linking table, the "Copy" table, is created to solve this many-to-many relationship (see Figure 3.15).

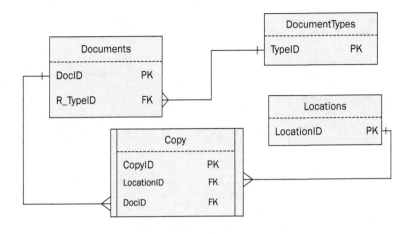

Figure 3.15 ER Diagram for Documentation Database

Normalization

Consistency is very important in a database design. In order to maintain consistency, we will introduce a new concept: Normalization. It is a systematic way of ensuring that a database structure is suitable for general-purpose querying and free of certain undesirable characteristics that could lead to a loss of data integrity. Normalization in relational data modeling is the process of decomposing large tables into smaller ones in order to eliminate redundant data and duplicate data and to avoid problems with inserting, updating, or deleting data. We will explain the process of normalization step by step below.

For example, Figure 3.16 shows a table for storing student information. When normalization rules have not yet been applied, this table is called a Zero Form.

Name	Major	Program_Director	EmailAddress1	EmailAddress2
Tom	HCA	John	tom@uwm.edu	tom@yahoo.com
Mary	HCA	John	ma@uwm.edu	
Joan	CLS	Mike	jo@uwm.edu	jo@ieee.org

Figure 3.16. Zero Form

This table poses some problems. You can see some repeating columns in this table, such as "EmailAddress1" and "EmailAddress2." If a student has more than two emails, we cannot store that information. Adding columns to this table for one student with three emails could create other problems. We will start normalizing for consistency in the database design.

First Normal Forms

The first normalization rule is to eliminate repeating groups in individual tables. In the student table, we will keep only one column for email addresses. In addition, we hope to identify each set of related data with a key. In this case, we will add a student ID (unique, automatically incrementing integer value) into every record in this table (see Figure 3.17).

Introduction to Healthcare Information Technology (First Edition)

First Normal Form

S_ID	Name	Major	Program _Director	EmailAddress
1	Tom	HCA	John	tom@uwm.edu
1	Tom	HCA	John	tom@yahoo.com
2	Mary	HCA	John	ma@uwm.edu
3	Joan	CLS	Mike	jo@ieee.org
3	Joan	CLS	Mike	jo@uwm.edu

Figure 3.17. First Normal Form

We can see that there are data duplication problems in this table. This will cause trouble in updating records. We need to further normalize the table.

Second Normal Forms

In the second step, we will create separate tables for sets of values that apply to multiple records. One large table becomes two tables: A "Student" table and an "Email" table. We need to relate these two tables with a foreign key. Let recall the definition of a foreign key: It is a column that defines how tables relate to each other and refers to a primary key in another table. We always add the foreign key in the Many side table. In this case, one student has many email addresses, so the "Email" table will be the Many side table. "R_S_ID" in the "Email" table is a foreign key (see Figure 3.18). Now the second normal form looks much better and more consistent. The "Student" table still has some data-duplication issues in terms of "Major" and "Program Director." Let's continue to normalize it.

S_ID	Name	Major	Program_Director	
1	Tom	HCA	John	Student
2	Mary	HCA	John	
3	Joan	CLS	Mike	

E_ID	R_S_ID	EmailAddress	
1	1	tom@uwm.edu	Email
2	1	tom@yahoo.com	
3	2	ma@uwm.edu	
4	3	jo@ieee.org	
5	3	jo@uwm.edu	

Figure 3.18. Second Normal Form

Third Normal Forms

In the third step, we need to eliminate fields that do not directly depend on the primary key. In the "Student" table above, "Program Director" does not directly depend on the primary key, "Student ID." We need to further create separate tables for sets of values that apply to multiple records. In this case, we will create a new table, a "Major" table. One major has many students. The student table is a Many side table, so we will create a foreign key, "R_M_ID," to establish the relationship between the "Student" table and the "Major" table (see Figure 3.19). The third Normal Forms are good enough for data consistency.

Third Normal Form

Student

S_ID	Name	R_M_ID
1	Tom	1
2	Mary	1
3	Joan	2

Major

M_ID	Major	Program_Director
1	HCA	John
2	CLS	Mike

Email

Email_ID	R_S_ID	EmailAddress
1	1	tom@uwm.edu
2	1	tom@yahoo.com
3	2	ma@uwm.edu
4	3	jo@ieee.org
5	3	jo@uwm.edu

Figure 3.19. Third Normal Forms

In summary, we list the normalization rules as follow [1].

- Eliminate repeating groups in individual tables.
- Identify each set of related data with a key.
- Create separate tables for sets of values that apply to multiple records.
- Relate these tables with a foreign key.
- Eliminate fields that do not directly depend on the key.

Normalization is a process, and the only way to learn a process is to practice and practice again.

Reference

Hernandez, M. *Database Design for Mere Mortals: A Hands-on Guide to Relational Database Design*, 2nd edition. Boston: Addison-Wesley Longman Publishing Co., Inc. 2003.

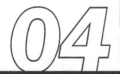

Medical Records and Coves

Why Do We Need Medical Records? [1]

The first reason is that medical records help healthcare workers recall information. It is the memory function of medical records. Physicians have short memories. Even if only one healthcare provider were involved, it is nearly impossible to remember exactly what each patient's problems were, what was done, and the patient's course of treatment without a written record. The second function of medical records is the communication function. As more and more healthcare providers are involved, the record becomes vital for communication among them. In the modern healthcare system, the communication function of medical records is more important than ever before.

Usage of Medical Records

Ideally, the primary use of medical records should be to assist in patient care. For example, the physician and the patient collaborated in making healthcare decisions for the patient. They decide on diagnostic efforts to be made and treatments to be used. The information in the medical records is vital to the success of this process.

Actually, there are many other reasons to create medical records, such as financial, legal, or operational reasons. Let's go through those secondary uses of medical records as follows: (1) Medical records are designed for billing for services. Currently healthcare organizations are still operating under the fee-for-service model. In medical records, procedures are documented in a certain way for billing purposes. (2) Physicians want to use medical records as essential evidence in court to protect themselves if there are potential malpractice legal defenses. (3) Besides physicians, people who have authority in hospitals, such as administrators, want to manage the hospitals to continue the business. They want to do basic administration work, quality review (statistics on performance, etc.), facilities/staff planning, etc. Medical records are designed for and used by administrators, too. (4) Governments also have power and want some information from medical records, such as infectious diseases, etc. This is another secondary use of medical records: Reporting to public health officials. (5) Some hospitals are teaching hospitals and have educational needs, so their medical records include some educational cases or functions. (6) Every year some medical research funds or grants are used to support clinical research projects, which use medical records. Unfortunately, patients do not have a lot of influence on the design of medical records. Hopefully, consumer health needs will pressure the improvement of medical-records design so that as citizens or patients, we can use medical records in a more friendly and convenient way in the future.

In short, medical-records design must first make sure that it helps in the care of the patient. It must not be constructed with administrative convenience first in mind or as a derivative of administrative paperwork.

Medical Data

Medical data has various formats. Some medical variables can be continuously monitored, such as ECG, blood pressure or respiratory frequency, etc. Some medical data are sampled, such as temperature and blood chemistry. Some parts of medical notes are free text to describe observations or interventions while some parts of medical notes can be coded, such as color, pain, position, drugs, anesthesia, etc. Now let's discuss the coding in medical records next. A code is something substituted for something else.

Why Do We Need Codes?

A word may have more than one meaning, so we create codes to increase precision in communication. In medical fields codes are used to obscure meaning to protect the privacy of the physician or patient. These days, computers are widely used, and codes can shorten information and facilitate its handling by electronic means.

How to Code (Classify) Data

Being able to classify or code objects is a useful skill. First, you need to list attributes of the object. Second, you will rank them based on the users' requirements (see Figure 4.1). Each of these aspects (attributes) can be used for a different ordering (called axis). Multiaxial classifications use several orderings simultaneously.

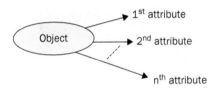

Figure 4.1 Classification

The only way to learn a skill is to practice and practice again. Let's try an exercise. For example, in order to design a web page for a used car dealer, we need to classify or code cars to help customers search. First, we can list all attributes of cars as follows:

- Type
- Year
- Make
- Model
- Color (Features)
- Mileage
- Price

• Miles Per Gallon (MPG)

Secondly, based on the customers' requirements analysis, we may rank those attributes as follows:

1. Make
2. Type
3. Model
4. Features
5. MPG
6. Mileage
7. Price
8. Year

The primary attribute will be the first level of axis and will be the first "tab name" or the top "pickup list name." For example, look at the user interface of a used car dealer website in Figure 4.2.

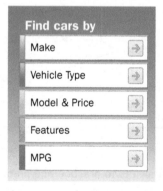

Figure 4.2. The Screen Copy of a Car Dealer Website

The ranking of attributes will be the structure of a classification or coding system. It will be decided based on the main purposes/objectives of the coding. Sometime, it may be arbitrary and created by classification/coding committees or workgroups.

Let's practice on an example in the healthcare field. In order to document diseases, we need to create a coding system for diseases. First, we need to list all attributes of diseases, such as anatomic location, etiology, morphology, dysfunction, etc. Second, based on the goals of the coding (clinical uses or public-health uses), we will rank the attributes and decide the structures of multiaxial classifications for diseases.

After we learn how to create a coding system, you may feel more comfortable understanding current medical codes. For example, ICD is an International Classification of Diseases (ICD), which was designed by the World Health Organization as a way to compare health statistics (e.g. mortality statistics) internationally. ICD is not classification of diseases but rather a classification of persons. It has variable multiaxial classifications, so it takes the various attributes of a case into account in deciding categories (see Figure 4.3). ICD solved the problem of collecting groups of cases for retrieval.

S55.11   Laceration of radial artery at forearm level
          S55.111   Laceration ...right arm
          S55.112   ... left arm
          S55.119   ... unspecified arm

Figure 4.3 ICD

Medical Codes

In this chapter, we will introduce some medical codes commonly used in medical documents. It will be helpful for you to understand coding in medical records. The coding system abbreviations will be discussed one by one.

ICD: International Classification of Diseases (ICD) was designed by World Health Organization. The primary use of ICD is international health statistics. There are modifications for clinical use after the sixth version of ICD, such as ICD-7-CM or ICD-10-CM. In addition, there are procedure classifications, such as ICD-10-PCS (Procedure Coding System). Some codes are designed for specific domains, such as ICD-O for oncology.

DRG: Diagnosis Related Groups (DRG) refers to the International Refined Diagnosis Related groupings, as developed by 3M. It is designed for budgeting, such as cost and length of stay. Cost is the total value of all activities for the encounter, as per the Fee-for-Service Basic Product Price List, including all drugs and medical devices, irrespective of whether the service is covered by the payer.

CPT: Current Procedural Terminology (CPT) is a medical code set maintained by the American Medical Association. It focuses on billing and reimbursement. CPT identifies the services provided and is used by insurance companies to determine how much physicians will be paid for their services.

ATC: Anatomic Therapeutic Chemical Code (drugs) (ACT) is used for the classification of active ingredients of drugs according to the organ or system on which they act and their therapeutic, pharmacological, and chemical properties. In this system, drugs are classified into groups at five different levels. The first level of the code indicates the anatomical main group and consists of one letter. For example, "C" refers to "cardiovascular system."

LOINC: Logical Observation Identifiers Names and Codes (LONIC) was created in 1994 by the Regenstrief Institute as a free, universal standard for laboratory and clinical observations to enable exchange of health information across different systems. LOINC is a code system used to identify test observations. It has been recognized as the preferred standard for coding testing and observations in HL7.

SNOMED: Systematized Nomenclature of Medicine SNOMED Clinical Terms (SNOMED CT) is a comprehensive, computerized healthcare terminology with the purpose of providing a common language across different providers and sites of care. As a core EHR terminology, SNOMED CT is essential for recording clinical data such as patient problem lists and family, medical, and social histories in electronic health records in a consistent, reproducible manner.

MeSH: Medical Subject Headings (MeSH) is a comprehensive controlled vocabulary for the purpose of indexing journal articles and books in the life sciences; it serves as a thesaurus that facilitates searching. Created and updated by the United States National Library of Medicine (NLM), it is used by the MEDLINE/PubMed article database and by NLM's catalog of book holdings. The subject headings in MeSH are arranged in a hierarchy.

What Are the Challenges of Coding for Computer Uses?

There are some challenges to designing a coding system for computer uses. For example, a computer is a machine and is sensitive to spelling errors. If you type one letter wrong or add a space in your codes, the computer may think it is a wrong answer. A computer may have trouble understanding the use of synonyms and lexical variations. Some codes, such as Read Clinical Classification (RCC), need to address those issues. Each code in RCC can be linked to a number of synonyms. Acronyms, eponyms, and abbreviations should be allowed for the use of natural language processing by computer.

In general, some standards dictate how information is communicated among humans, such as healthcare consumers, providers, payers, and other interested parties. For example, ICD and SNOMED are designed for humans to process information while there are some standards which dictate how information is communicated electronically between machines, such as HL7 or DICOM.

What Is HIPAA?

The Health Insurance Portability and Accountability Act (HIPAA) is a federal law intended to protect health information. HIPAA will have a profound impact on overall healthcare industry electronic communications and transactions. HIPAA has three major components as follows: "Transactions and Code Sets," "Security Regulations," and "Privacy Regulations." HIPAA includes the standards for communicating between healthcare providers and payers (see Figure 4.4).

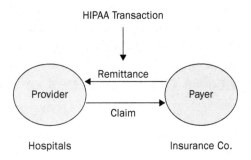

Figure 4.4 Figure 4.4 HIPAA Messages

HIPAA privacy regulations cover privacy and confidentiality issues. Privacy is the ability to control what, when, and with whom your personal information is shared. It is the right of an individual to be left alone. HIPAA defines 18 "Protected Health Information" (PHI) items, such as individually identifiable information (names). Confidentiality is the act of limiting disclosure of personal information which has been entrusted to another with the confidence that unauthorized disclosure will not occur. HIPAA Security Regulations provide requirements for information system security in detail.

Reference

Slee, Virgil, Debora Slee, and H. Joachim Schmidt. *The Endangered Medical Record: Ensuring Its Integrity in the Age of Informatics*, St. Paul, MN: Tringa Press, 2000.

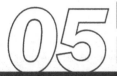

Electronic Medical Records

What Are the Limitations of Paper-based Medical Records?

Paper-based medical records have certain limitations. For example, some physicians' handwriting is hard to read. Another problem is that paper-based records cannot be easily searched, and they are difficult to access in more than one place. Most paper-based medical records are stored in folders in cabinets. This may cause a security problem because access to these records cannot be easily tracked, and the records may not be secure from unauthorized uses and users. In the first chapter, we already introduced the computer and know what computers are useful for, such as record storage and fast computation. Current information technology provides databases and the Internet for the processing of medical information. Naturally, we start using Electronic Medical Records (EMR).

What Are Electronic Medical Records (EMR)?

EMR is used loosely today to describe many medical records kept in digital format on a computer with constant instantaneous access via computer terminal. Also it is called Computer-based Patient Records (CPR).

The Primary Goal of EMR Design

In Chapter 4, we discussed the primary and secondary uses of medical records. To design electronic medical records, we should focus on the primary uses of EMR. EMR must help patient care. Healthcare providers are essential to the EMR design. EMR must not interfere with patient care and should not increase workloads on the part of the physician to process information. Healthcare providers should not be forced to change their work habits.

Indexes of EMR

For different purposes or situations, medical data can be structured/viewed in different formats (indexes), such as time-oriented, source-oriented, and problem-oriented.

Time-oriented Format

The diagnostic-therapeutic loop has different stages, such as observations, decisions, and interventions. For example, if a series of events happened, as follows (see Figure 5.1), T1 can be the first visit, T2 is the follow-up visit, T3 is another follow-up visit, T4 can be the hospital admission, T5 is the hospital discharge, and T6 may be the follow-up visit after that. Each event contains different actions and related data elements.

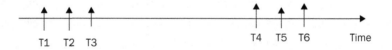

Figure 5.1 Time-oriented Data Format

It is very natural and intuitive to organize medical information following a time sequence, such as this example of time-oriented medical records.

Introduction to Healthcare Information Technology (First Edition)

Feb 21, 2016:

Shortness of breath, cough, and fever. Very dark feces. Exam: RR 150/90, pulse 95/min, Temp: 39.3C, abdomen not tender. Present medication 64 mg Aspirin per day. Probably acute bronchitis, possibly complicated by cardiac decompensation. Bleeding possibly due to Aspirin. ESR 25 mm, Hb 7.8, occult blood feces +, Chest X-ray: no atelectasis. Medication: Amoxicillin caps 500mg twice daily, Aspirin reduce to 32 mg per day.

Mar 4, 2016:

No more cough, slight shortness of breath, normal feces. Exam: slight rhonchi, RR 160/95, pulse 82/min.

Source-oriented Format

In addition, we can organize the medical data based on the data source (location), such as the example of source-oriented medical records below.

Visits

Feb 21, 2016: Shortness of breath, cough, and fever. Very dark feces. Exam: RR 150/90, pulse 95/min, Temp: 39.3C, abdomen not tender. Present medication 64 mg Aspirin per day. Probably acute bronchitis, possibly complicated by cardiac decompensation. Bleeding possibly due to Aspirin. Medication: Amoxicillin caps 500mg twice daily, Aspirin Reduce to 32 mg per day.

Mar 4, 2016: No more cough, slight shortness of breath, normal feces. Exam: slight rhonchi, RR 160/95, pulse 82/min.

Laboratory tests

Feb 21, 2016: ESR 25 mm, Hb 7.8, occult blood feces + X-rays

Feb 21, 2016: Chest X-ray: no atelectasis

Problem-oriented Format

Some clinical notes are designed in problem-oriented formats, such as S.O.A.P notes. S.O.A.P. is an acronym for a specific style of documentation. Each letter represents a section of the note as follows:

Subjective: Information that the physician gains from interviewing or talking with the patient, a family member, a significant other, or any individual who provides information that is pertinent to the care of the patient.

Objective: Information that the physician acquires from the physical examination (includes observations, specific measurements, special tests, etc.). "O" also includes treatment administered to the patient and the patient's performance of the treatment.

Assessment: This is the physician's "opinion section" of the note. It contains the physician's professional opinion of what is going on with the patient, the physician's assessment of the patient's condition and/or progress, the physician's prognosis, treatment goals, and the physician's recommendations.

Plan: Reflects future treatments, interventions, or actions by the physician.

A list of problems in medical records could be an ideal index to retrieve all related information around one patient problem. Here is an example of problem-oriented medical records:

Problem 1: Acute bronchitis

Feb 21, 2016: S: Shortness of breath, cough, and fever.
    O: pulse 95/min, Temp: 39.3C, ESR 25 mm, Hb 7.8, occult blood feces +,
    Chest X-ray: no atelectasis
    A: Acute bronchitis,
    P: Amoxicillin caps 500mg twice daily

Mar4, 2016: S: No more cough, slight shortness of breath

O: slight rhonchi, pulse 82/min.

Problem 2: Shortness of breath

Feb 21, 2016: S: Shortness of breath
    O: RR 150/90, Chest X-ray: no atelectasis
    A: possibly complicated by cardiac decompensation.

Mar 4, 2016: S: slight shortness of breath
    O: RR 160/95,
    A: No decompensation

Problem 3: Dark feces...

Integrated Data Format

Today when we design new electronic medical records, we have more choices, such as multimedia (videos, images, graphics, etc.). We can design integrated formats/views of medical records. In Figure 5.2 the horizontal is a time line, and the vertical is a problem list. Different colors are used to represent different locations (sources). The integrated format can present more information in a graphic chart and potentially be more user friendly.

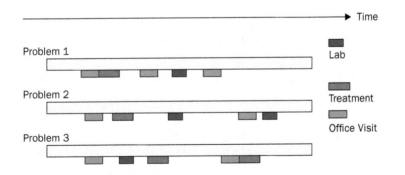

Figure 5.2 Integrated EMR

What Key Attributes should EMR Have?

When we purchase a car, we need to know key features of the car, such as engine power, safety, miles per gallon, etc. Similarly, before we buy a computer, we want to find out how fast the computer is (CPU frequency in GHz) and how large the main memory is (RAM size in GB). In order to purchase expensive electronic medical records systems, healthcare providers also need to know key attributes of EMR.

"Key Attributes"[1]

A list of key attributes of Computer-based Patient Records (CPR) has been developed by The Institute of Medicine (IOM). We will discuss them one by one as follows:

1. Offers a problem list.
It identifies a problem list that can serve as a good index to retrieve a patient's information in medical records.

2. Has ability to measure health status and functional levels.

   It is required to prioritize patients in emergency rooms (ER) or monitor patients in intensive care units (ICU).

3. Can document clinical reasoning and rationale.

   It will help healthcare providers to communicate efficiently about patients' diagnoses and treatments.

4. Is longitudinal and has timely linkages with other patient records.

   Time is a critical attribute for health care. All vital signs and patient information should be recorded with time value. The central database in an electronic medical records system should be designed to store time-oriented variables. For example, when we record a patient's temperature, we also need to know when the temperature was measured, such as early morning or late afternoon.

5. Guaranteed confidentiality, privacy, and audit trails.

   This feature emphasizes compliance with HIPAA regulations about privacy and security.

6. Offers continuous access for authorized users.

   One of requirements for information system design is that it should provide services twenty-four hours per day and seven days per week to maintain the business continuity.

7. Supports simultaneous multiple-user views into the CPR.

   The system should be robust to support concurrent uses and have mirror servers to handle large influxes of user requests.

8. Supports timely access to local and remote information resources.

   The EMR system should be web-based and provide tele-medicine functions.

9. Facilitates clinical problem solving.

   The EMR system should provide Computer Decision Support System (CDSS) components to support medical decision making.

10. Supports direct data entry by physicians.

    The EMR system should include computerized physician order entry (CPOE) components.

11. Supports practitioners in measuring or managing costs and improving quality.

The EMR system will meet requirements for quality control and administration.

12. Has flexibility to support existing or evolving needs of clinical specialties.

To meeting the changes in the future, the EMR system design should be robust and have multiple layers to provide data independence and flexibility for changes.

Meaningful Uses Standards

In 2008, a financial crisis broke out. In 2009, the American Recovery and Reinvestment Act (ARRA) authorized the Centers for Medicare and Medicaid Services (CMS) to provide a reimbursement incentive for physician and hospital providers who are successful in becoming "meaningful users" of an electronic health record (EHR), and in February, 2009, ARRA was signed into law. The Office of the National Coordinator for Health Information Technology (ONC) determines whether EHR use is "meaningful." This is the new standard for EMR: Meaningful Uses. Updated information about meaningful uses can be found at the website of the Center for Medicare and Medicaid Services (CMS).

Meaningful Uses standards define key functions of the EMR system. Stage 2 core and menu objectives for eligible professionals are listed as follows [2].

17 Core Objectives:

1. Use computerized provider order entry (CPOE) for medication, laboratory, and radiology orders
2. Generate and transmit permissible prescriptions electronically (eRx)
3. Record demographic information
4. Record and chart changes in vital signs
5. Record smoking status for patients 13 years old or older

6. Use clinical decision support to improve performance on high-priority health conditions
7. Provide patients the ability to view online, download, and transmit their health information
8. Provide clinical summaries for patients for each office visit
9. Protect electronic health information created or maintained by the Certified EHR Technology
10. Incorporate clinical lab-test results into Certified EHR Technology
11. Generate lists of patients by specific conditions to use for quality improvement, reduction of disparities, research, or outreach
12. Use clinically relevant information to identify patients who should receive reminders for preventive/follow-up care
13. Use certified EHR technology to identify patient-specific education resources
14. Perform medication reconciliation
15. Provide summary of care record for each transition of care or referral
16. Submit electronic data to immunization registries
17. Use secure electronic messaging to communicate with patients on relevant health information

3 of 6 Menu Objectives:

1. Submit electronic syndromic surveillance data to public health agencies
2. Record electronic notes in patient records
3. Imaging results accessible through CEHRT
4. Record patient family health history
5. Identify and report cancer cases to a state cancer registry
6. Identify and report specific cases to a specialized registry (other than a cancer registry)

Here are stage 2 core and menu objectives for eligible Hospitals [3].

16 Core Objectives:

1. Use computerized provider order entry (CPOE) for medication, laboratory, and radiology orders

2. Record demographic information
3. Record and chart changes in vital signs
4. Record smoking status for patients 13 years old or older
5. Use clinical decision support to improve performance on high-priority health conditions
6. Provide patients the ability to view online, download, and transmit their health information within 36 hours after discharge.
7. Protect electronic health information created or maintained by the Certified EHR Technology
8. Incorporate clinical lab-test results into Certified EHR Technology
9. Generate lists of patients by specific conditions to use for quality improvement, reduction of disparities, research, or outreach
10. Use certified EHR technology to identify patient-specific education resources and provide those resources to the patient if appropriate
11. Perform medication reconciliation
12. Provide summary of care record for each transition of care or referral
13. Submit electronic data to immunization registries
14. Submit electronic data on reportable lab results to public health agencies
15. Submit electronic syndromic surveillance data to public health agencies
16. Automatically track medications with an electronic medication administration record (eMAR)

3 of 6 Menu Objectives:

1. Record whether a patient 65 years old or older has an advance directive
2. Record electronic notes in patient records
3. Imaging results accessible through CEHRT
4. Record patient family health history
5. Generate and transmit permissible discharge prescriptions electronically (eRx)
6. Provide structured electronic lab results to ambulatory providers

Computerized Physician Order Entry (CPOE)

In Meaningful Uses Standards, CPOE is one of key functions for EMR. It will allows physicians to directly enter orders, such as medication orders, admission/discharge/transfer orders, nursing orders, laboratory orders, radiology orders, dietary orders, consults and procedures orders, and others.

Why Do We Need CPOE?

CPOE can help healthcare systems to reduce medical errors. For example, some physicians' handwriting can be hard to read. CPOE can improve care quality. For example, clinical guidelines can be integrated into CPOE workflow and provide updated, standardized, best practice information to physicians at the point of care. CPOE can reduce costs. For example, physicians can have medication orders using CPOE, and the electronic prescriptions can be efficiently shared with the pharmacy and patient. In addition, related insurance coverage information about medications will be available for decision making.

What Are the Challenges of CPOE?

In the past, paper-based order sets have had different structures, various quality, inconsistencies, different coverages, and out-of-date information. We do not want to simply re-implement those existing issues. Actually, CPOE provides an opportunity to change. The challenge is that CPOE require changes in provider workflow. Implementing CPOE involves a great deal of change. Success of CPOE design requires changing clinical processes and practices, which in turn requires addressing a myriad of details concerning how work actually gets done and being flexible and responsive to issues identified during rollout. CPOE may increase the time providers spend on orders. The requirement for CPOE is high, so it really is a challenging task to design CPOE.

What Are the Requirements of CPOE Design?

For health care, the first requirement of CPOE design is accuracy. Accuracy of 95% is not good enough; 100% should be the goal. At the same time, pickup lists in CPOE orders should be complete, consistent, and easy to use. In design, there are tradeoffs among key attributes of CPOE. For example, when we have a complex hierarchy to obtain information necessary to process the request accurately, CPOE may not be simple and easy to use. When we have more prerequisites for accuracy, it will be less easy to use. A better design meets all requirements. For example, a complete list of test orders can be a long pick-up list presented alphabetically on multiple screens. Based on the statistics analysis of old test orders, we can find the most frequently ordered tests. We may put those orders at the top of pick-up list to be shown in the first screen.

Computer Decision Support System (CDSS)

In health care, there are many uncertainties. For example, a clinician usually cannot be certain what a finding implies about the patient's true state, and the clinician may say that a disease is "possibly" present. We can use probability, which is an alternative method of expressing uncertainty. For example, if a patient has a prior probability for a specific disease, which is a description of what is known about a variable in the absence of some evidence, and a test related to a hypothesis of the disease is performed, a post-test probability, shown in Figure 5.3, can be obtained.

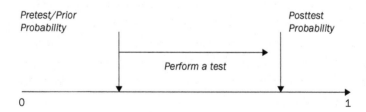

Figure 5.3 Use probability to describe uncertainty

Why Is Clinical Decision Making Complex?

Clinical decision making is difficult because tests are not perfect. Normally, specificity and sensitivity are used to describe the accuracy of available diagnostic tests. The natural history of the disease is complex and various. Also, the effects of treatment in an individual cannot be certain because normally only data about average effects of an intervention in a group (population) as a whole is available. Erroneous observations, inaccurate recording of clinical findings, or misinterpretation of the data can be contributing factors as well. These days, an integrated decision will be made among physicians and patients together, so patient preferences will be considered. For example, patients may choose maximizing life expectancy (e.g., live longer with pain) or optimizing quality of life (e.g., live better without pain). In reality, financial concerns (minimizing the resources required) will be another factor in clinical decision making.

CDSS Applications

CDSS can be applied into many areas, such as decision support on drug orders, laboratory testing, or radiology procedures. There are many specific CDSS applications for drugs. For example, computers can help healthcare providers conduct drug name checking, patient drug allergies checking, drug-to-drug interaction checking, drug-cost display, guided-dosing calculation, etc. In addition, CDSS can be applied to diagnostic tests. For instance, CDSS can help diagnosis or problem-based order sets, provide suggestions for alternate tests, list prerequisite or subsequent tests, do redundant test checks, display costs, and display recent results. In many areas in hospitals, computers can provide decision supports. For example, computer systems can conduct default administration routing implement protocol or diagnosis-based therapy, and provide time-based checks to ensure optimum timing and duration. In those CDSS applications, computers generate reminders, suggestions, or alerts to help physicians' decision making at the point of care (see Figure 5.4).

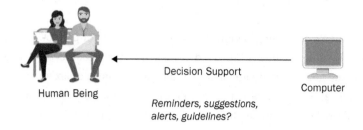

Figure 5.4 Decision Support

Clinicians Acceptance of CDSS

One challenge to implementing CDSS is clinicians' acceptance (see Figure 5.5). Many physicians still have strong resistance toward using CDSS in complex decisions. For example, clinicians may have strong beliefs about a medication, ignoring the suggestion of others by CDSS. However, many clinicians do not have strong feelings about the changing direction in other contexts. For instance, many clinicians will accept the computer's suggestion of dose, route, or frequency of a medication.

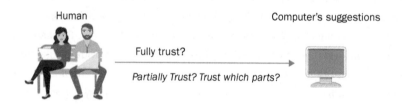

Figure 5.5 Clinicians Acceptance of CDSS

Implementation Issues of CDSS

There are two ways to use CDSS, passive and active. In the passive mode, CDSS may have low usage. In order to have CDSS in active mode, the

Introduction to Healthcare Information Technology (First Edition)

timing of triggers must be identified. For example, the guidelines can be displayed to the user at the time the clinician is in the process of ordering a medication or treatment, such as by a pop-up window at the right moment. In order to design active CDSS, it is critical for designers to fully understand clinician workflows and identify the timing of intervention.

CDSS should be easy to use. For example, a guideline can be presented on a single screen, and it may require substantial condensation and simplification. Simple interventions work best, so we need to design friendly CDSS to convince clinicians to use it, and provide more information only when clinicians really need it.

References

Institute of Medicine (Corporate Author), Elaine B. Steen (Editor), Don E. Detmer (Editor). *The Computer-Based Patient Record: An Essential Technology for Health Care*. National Academy Press. January 15, 1997.

Center of Medicare Service (CMS). "Eligible Professional (EP) Meaningful Use Core and Menu Measures." www.cms.gov. https://www.cms.gov/regulations-and-guidance/legislation/ehrincentiveprograms/downloads/stage2_meaningfulusespecsheet_tablecontents_eps.pdf (accessed June 8, 2016).

Center of Medicare Service (CMS). "Eligible Hospital and Critical Access Hospital (CAH) Meaningful Use Core and Menu Objectives." www.cms.gov. https://www.cms.gov/regulations-and-guidance/legislation/ehrincentiveprograms/downloads/stage2_meaningfulusespecsheet_tablecontents_eligiblehospitals_cahs.pdf (accessed June 8, 2016).

Credits

Relational Data Model: Physical Design

Physical design is to decide how the logical design is to be physically implemented in the target database management system (DBMS). DBMS is a software program you use to create, maintain, modify, and manipulate a database.

The first task is to select a DBMS based on your project's needs. If your project has high-end mission-critical applications with a large budget, in general, we can choose from the market leaders, and that means one of the big three: Oracle, IBM DB2, or Microsoft SQL Server. Those general-purpose designed DBMSs are robust and have many utilities for users to explore, such as data-mining packages or geographic utilities. Unfortunately, those DBMS are complex and expensive. For a low-budget project, we also can choose open-source DBMS, like MySQL or PostgreSQL. They are free and simple. Sometimes, they are good enough for most lower-end, web-based development projects. In this course, we choose Microsoft Access as DBMS, because it is a database management system for personal use, and it is easy to learn. It supports graphic user interfaces (GUI) to create and modify a database.

What Does DBMS Provide?

DBMS is a powerful middleware (system software). It supports concurrent control to provide concurrent access of data to multiple users. It is the middle layer in the multiple-layer system architecture, so it provide the data independence, which is to hide the details of the storage structure from user applications. The DBMS supports SQL or related languages, so users can have more efficient data access and data can be shared. For data integrity and security, DBMS provides capabilities for defining and enforcing the integrity and security constraints. It can control redundancy, and inconsistency can be avoided. DBMS can restrict unauthorized access. In addition, it provides backup and recovery. DBMS can manage users and their privileges. Because DBMS provides standardized application interfaces for developers, it can reduce application development time.

Business Rules and Data Integrity

In physical design, we need to address "Business Rules" and "Data Integrity." We will introduce those concepts to you and discuss some implementation of data integrity.

"Business rules" specify conditions and relationships that must always be true or must always be false. When we manipulate data, such as inserting, updating, deleting, and viewing data, specific conditions must be met. For example, if your application applies new sales orders to the invoice file, a business rule should automatically check the customer's credit limit before accepting and inserting the sales order line items. Some business rules require us to validate data, such as, "the numeric field is really within range," and "the publisher identification does exist in the publishers file."

"Data integrity" refers to the completeness, accuracy, and consistency of data stored in a database. Often used as a proxy for "data quality," it overlaps with "database security" concepts, which refers to data encryption, data backup, access controls, input validation, data validation, etc. Business rules can overlap with "data integrity." For example, the business rules in a project may specify the requirements of controlling data security and providing referential integrity.

Implementation of Data Integrity

At the Table level, we can apply the primary keys to the table. Each row in a table should be identified by a unique identifier (primary key). The primary key (column) of the table cannot be null. By enforcing the primary keys in tables, we can make sure that there are no duplicate rows in a table.

At the Field level, we can validate data in the field specifications, such as data type (number, text, etc.), length, input mask, or display format.

At the Relationship level, we can enforce referential integrity constraints. Each value of the foreign key in one table must have a matching value in the referenced key in another table. Otherwise, it's called a "dangling reference," and the DBMS will provide error messages. For example, in a student class registration database (see Figure 6.1), the referential integrity constraint is maintaining data integrity for tables in this database, such as "Classes," "Students," and "Registration."

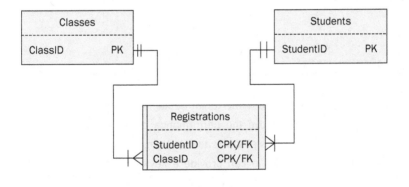

Figure 6.1 ER Diagram for Registration System

Figure 6.2 demonstrates the referential integrity. To insert records, the correct sequence is to insert records to "one" tables ("Classes" table and "Students" table) first; then you can insert records to "Many" tables later ("Registration" table). It will be appropriate to first delete records from "Many" tables ("Registration" table); then you can delete records from

"One" tables ("Classes" table and "Students" table). If you delete records in the "Class" or "Student" tables first, the DBMS will provide error messages to you: "You have violated the referential integrity."

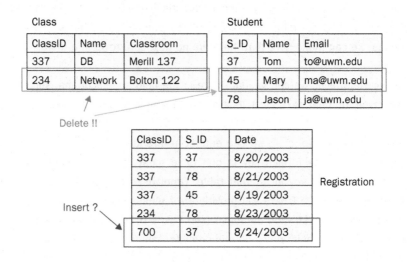

Figure 6.2 Demonstration of Referential Integrity

Performance Tuning

In the physical design, we want to introduce the "performance tuning" concept, which is to improve the performance of the database, such as making it faster. For example, if a reader is trying to find a word in a book by examining each page, we can provide a keyword index in the back of the book, and it will significantly improve the performance of information retrieval, and that reader can complete the task in a much shorter time. It is the same idea that effective indexes are one of the best ways to improve performance in a database application. We can create indexes to improve query response time. However, indexing is a balancing act because when a query modifies the data in a table, the indexes on the data must change also.

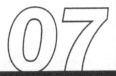

Database Design: Case Study

To design a database in a short time, students are requested to identify a topic with which they are very familiar. They understand all the related information about this topic, so it will save a lot of time for data collection of user requirements, such as user interviews. In previous semesters, students chose topics directly related to their lives, such as personal toy collections, sports, places where they have been customers, such as hair salons, or working experiences, such as tutoring.

Personal Toy Collection

The purpose of the toy database is to maintain an accurate record of the types of toys in the collection, the location of those toys, the manufacturer of the toys, the series the toys are from, and the description of the toys to determine which ones are still needed to complete the collections and track the ones that are already owned. One person can have many toys. A collection of toys can have many types. Each toy has a specific location, description, and name. Each group of toys can have a different manufacturer. Each toy is from a different series.

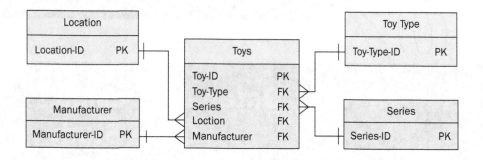

Figure 7.0a ER for Toy Collection

Tutoring Records

The purpose of the tutoring database is to maintain an accurate record of the tutoring information needed for each student, a record of their contract with the company and what it entails, a record of the type of classes the student seeks assistance in, a record of the teachers in the company and the subjects they specialize in, and to document and keep track of the performance/progress of each student. One student may need help in many different academic subjects, not just one. Therefore, since one tutor specializes in one subject, a student can have many different tutors. This system also keeps record of the student's performance report.

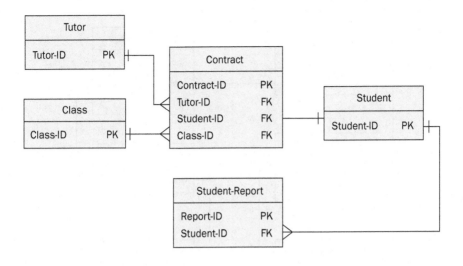

Figure 7.0b ER for Tutoring System

Volleyball Season

The purpose of the volleyball database is to get an accurate record of the games in a season. This includes the number of matches played in each game with wins and losses, players and their full name with their position, the teams playing in the game, the number of players on each team and their team name, and the statistics of all the players. One game has many matches. There are many teams in a game. One team has many players. Each player has many statistics. One game has many matches. One team can play many games. Each game involves two teams. One team has many players. Each player has many performance reports with statistics, such as number of kills in a game.

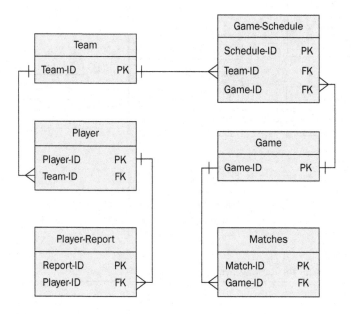

Figure 7.0c ER for Volleyball Tournaments

UWM Planetarium Event Reservations

The UWM Planetarium would like to record what schools/private groups are reserving the facility. The purpose of this database is to maintain the school/private group information as well as the reservation information. The Planetarium would also like to record which staff member is monitoring these events. One school/organization can book many events at different times. One event must have at least one staff member monitoring the event. The staff member can join many events. One event can have many activities scheduled. Many events have similar activities.

Introduction to Healthcare Information Technology (First Edition)

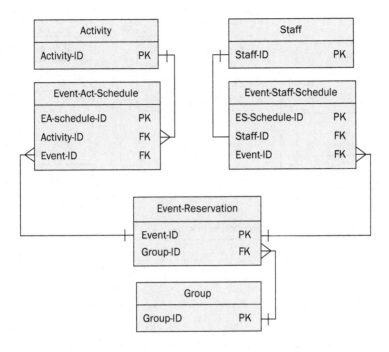

Figure 7.0d ER for Event Reservation

Hair Salon Appointments

The purpose of a hair salon database, is to maintain data the reception-ist will use to schedule appointments and record services provided to clients. Each store has many stylists. Each stylist will have appointments. Each appointment specifies a service type. Customers can make many appointments.

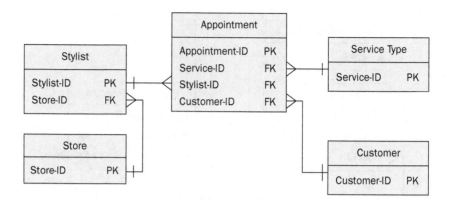

Figure 7.0e ER for Hair Salon Appointments

Boat Rental

For people who would like to have occasional fun on the water when the weather is nice, renting a boat may make more sense financially versus buying a boat. A boat rental company can have a variety of different boats and multiple locations. It can also have multiple customers per day, so the company can have many different reservations. The purpose of this boat rental database is to provide an accurate record for the company regarding the location, the boat, the customer, the rental agreement, and the insurance. By having an accurate record of these things, the company can stay organized in order to provide an easy, enjoyable experience for the customer along with tracking any sort of damage done to the boats. One location can have many boats.

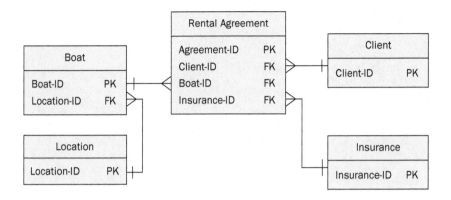

Figure ER for Boat Rental

One Contact Person can book many events. One Contact Person can only be a reference to one school/organization. One Event must have at least one staff member monitoring the event. One Event can have many or zero activities scheduled.

Data Model Patterns

You may find that "Appointment ER" and "Rental Agreement ER" are similar. This is a data model pattern, which describes recurring solutions to common problems, such as appointments, reservations, agreements, or contracts. If we can identify the pattern, we already have the basic elements of any similar situations. Understanding those similarities gives us a starting model. We can adjust it as necessary to match the specific circumstances. All we need to do is to continue to add more model patterns to our toolbox.

Network

Network Model

A network model includes a group of nodes, like a tangled web (see Figure 8.1). Those nodes can be persons or computers. In this model, any nodes can point to any other nodes, and there are peer-to-peer relationships. It is easy to set links between nodes, so it's hard to control these networks.

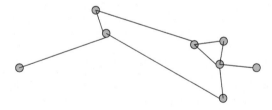

Figure 8.1 Network Model

To study a network, we need to address two questions as follows:
- ❏ How to identify each node? (Identification Issue)
- ❏ How to communicate between two nodes? (Network Communication Rules Issue)

Network Identification

How are you (a person) identified in the human network? You have a name, a mailing address, a phone number, and perhaps an email address. To reach you, we can call you, email you, or mail a letter to you. How is a computer identified in the classroom? Does this PC have a name? The short answer is yes, and the PC name is globally unique. What does the PC name look like? Actually, the computer has a Network Interface Card (NIC), and it has a Media Access Control Address (MAC), such as 03-A1-22-70-4F-07. It is a long number (48 bits) and is a physical address of a computer in the network.

Besides the MAC (physical address) uniquely associated with hardware, a computer can have logical names. We can create a logical address: Internet Address (IP). The IP address (logical) and MAC address (physical) are mapped to each other. There are related rules (ARP or RARP) to match them (see Figure 8.2). ARP is Address Resolution Protocol, and RARP is Reverse Address Resolution Protocol.

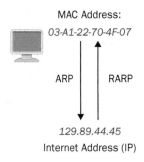

Figure 8.2 Network Identifications

Every node on an internet has a unique IP address, and it has a dotted-decimal notation, such as 129.89.44.46. It is also a long number with 32 bits. Each IP address is hierarchically organized and includes the network number and host number in it. The Internet Network Information Center (InterNIC) has the central authority to assign only network numbers. Local network administrators in a network will manage the host number within the local network. There are three types of IP addresses: Unicast address is destined for a single host; Broadcast address is destined for all hosts on a given network; and Multicast address is destined for a set of hosts that belong to a multicast group.

Domain Name Server (DNS)

Humans work best using the name of a host instead of a dotted-decimal IP address. There are maps between IP addresses and hostnames. Domain Name Servers (DNS) is a distribution database storing IP addresses and hostnames. Each time the application first looks up the IP address corresponding to a given hostname from DNS. For example, if the UWM D2L course website address is d2l.uwm.edu (hostname), the DNS will find that the related IP address for this course website at UWM is 129.89.70.157.

Network Communication Rules

In the human network, we use different languages to communicate among ourselves. In a computer network, we need to develop network communication rules, which are called Networking Protocols (see Figure 8.3).

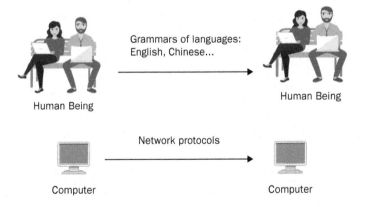

Figure 8.3 Network Protocols

Computers are machines. We have to break complex tasks into smaller one for computers to handle. We use abstractions to hide the complexity of networks, and abstraction naturally leads to layering of networks. Networking protocols are normally developed in layers. Each layer is a response to a different facet of the communications. A protocol suite is the combination of different protocols at various layers (see Figure 8.4), including the hardware layer, the host-to-host activity layer, the process-to-process communication layer, and the application-programs layer.

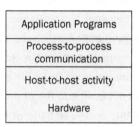

Figure 8.4 Multilayers of Network Protocols

Each protocol object has two different interfaces (see Figure 8.5). Service interface defines operations within this protocol, and peer-to-peer interface defines messages exchanged with peers. The protocol consists of a specification of peer-to-peer interface and a module that implements this interface.

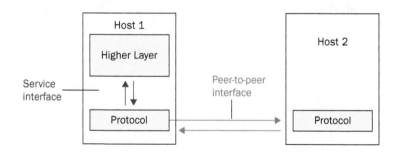

Figure 8.5 Two Faces of Each Network Protocol

A protocol suite, TCP/IP, will be discussed in detail because it is widely accepted and used these days. TCP/IP is the combination of different protocols at four layers (see Figure 8.6), which are the link layer, the network layer, the transport layer, and the application layer.

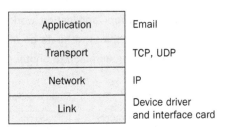

Application	Email
Transport	TCP, UDP
Network	IP
Link	Device driver and interface card

Figure 8.6 TCP/IP Protocol Suite

The link (data-link, network interface) layer includes the device driver in the operating system and the corresponding network interface card in the computer.

The network layer handles the movement of packets around the network, including routing packets. IP is Internet Protocol. ICMP is Internet Control Message Protocol. IGMP is Internet Group Management Protocol.

The transport layer provides a flow of data between hosts. TCP (Transmission Control Protocol) provides a reliable flow of data between hosts. (Acknowledging received packets, setting timeouts to make certain the other end acknowledges packets that are sent, and so on.) The way of communication in TCP is just like making a phone call. It is widely used for financial transaction applications with high security requirements. UDP (User Datagram Protocol) provides a much simpler service to the application layer. There is no guarantee that the data will reach the other end. The way of communication in UDP is like sending a letter. For example, UDP can be used for video applications and provides relatively fast performance.

The application layer handles the details of the particular application. For example, Telnet can provide a remote login. FTP is the File Transfer

Protocol. SMTP is the Simple Mail Transfer Protocol for electronic mail. HL7 is a health level 7 protocol.

Network Applications - Email

We will demonstrate how the network application works through TCP/IP layers (see Figure 8.7). In this example, two hosts on a local network are running SMTP. One person is sending an email to another person.

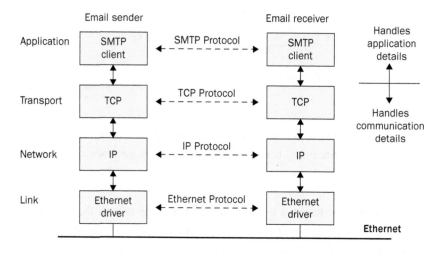

Figure 8.7 Network Applications: Email

Encapsulation of Data

When data is sent down the protocol stack through each layer, it is sent as a stream of bits across the network. Each layer adds information to the data by adding headers to the data that is received (see Figure 8.8). They are application data, TCP segment, IP datagram, and Ethernet frame.

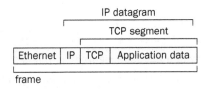

Figure 8.8 Encapsulation Data

How to Set Up a Local Network

In order to set up a local network, we need to know some basic network physical layouts and network devices. First, we will introduce some network physical layouts, also called Network Topology.

Bus Topology or Linear Bus

The simplest form of networking is a bus topology (see Figure 8.9), and it is the least expensive to implement. A single cable connects all computers in the network in a single line without any active electronics to amplify or modify the signal. This bus must be terminated at each end. It is a passive topology because each computer only monitors the signals on the bus.

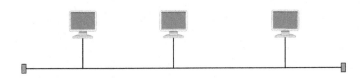

Figure 8.9 Linear bus

Star Topology

Star topology requires the purchase of a hub, so all devices on the network are connected directly to a hub (see Figure 8.10). It is easy to troubleshoot because each device can be individually unplugged from the hub.

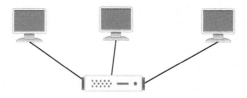

Figure 8.10 Star Topology

Variations of Star and Bus Topology

Actually, we can combine several hubs together and create a cascaded star topology (see Figure 8.11).

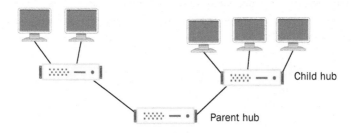

Child hub

Parent hub

Figure 8.11 Cascaded Star Topology

In addition, we can combine bus topology and star topology together and create a star-bus topology (see Figure 8.12).

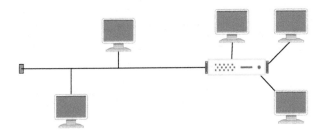

Figure 8.12 Star-bus Topology

Ring Topology

The ring topology is that all computers are connected by segments of cable in a ring fashion with no ends to the network (see Figure 8.13). The signal passes through each computer on the network and is reconditioned before being retransmitted. If any computer fails, then the entire network goes down.

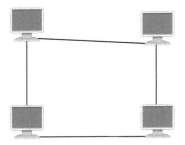

Figure 8.13 Ring Topology

Now, we can introduce some network devices, such as repeater, bridge, switch, and router. Repeaters are active devices that regenerate incoming signals. Signals are boosted as they pass through the repeaters (see Figure 8.14).

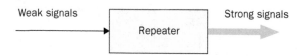

Weak signals   Strong signals

Repeater

Figure 8.14 Repeater

A bridge device is like a repeater device, but a bridge is more selective and passes only those signals targeted for a computer on the other side (see Figure 8.15). The bridge receives every packet on LAN A and LAN B. The bridge learns from packets which devices on the LAN require the information and builds a table with this information. Packets on LAN A addressed to devices on LAN A are discarded by the bridge since packets can be delivered in LAN without the help of bridge. Packets on LAN A addressed to devices on LAN B are retransmitted to LAN B for delivery.

A switch is a learning bridge with improved performance. It does not block broadcast packets. It can filter out traffic that isn't destined for a station on a given port so that the station sees less network traffic and can perform better.

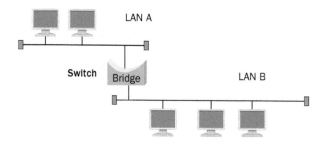

Figure 8.15 Bridge or Switch Device

A router is more intelligent than a switch, and it build tables of network locations (see Figure 8.16). A router can use algorithms to determine the most efficient path for sending a packet to any given network. Even if a particular network segment isn't directly attached to the router, the router knows the best way to send a packet to a device on that network.

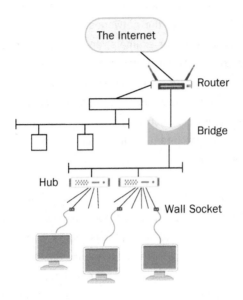

Figure 8.16 Router Device

In summary, those network devices/drivers work in different layers (see Figure 8.17). In the hardware layer, we have network devices, such as hub, repeater, and concentrator. In the network layer, we have more intelligent network devices, such as bridge, switch, and router.

Gateway	Application
	Transport
Bridge, switch, router	Network
Hub, repeater, concentrator	Link

Figure 8.17 Summary of Network Devices

Network Security

A network connects everyone together and becomes more and more important. We have to address the network-security issue. There are many network-security problems. For example, on the user side, a user may be careless in forgetting passwords or making errors for lost passwords. A network has multiple layers and can be complex, so network software may have security holes, such as inappropriately configured firewalls. In addition, natural disasters, such as flooding or fire, may destroy network devices. Hackers can also intentionally attack a system and steal information through the network.

We need to prepare security solutions for those threats. For example, we can deny physical access to areas containing key network resources. Surveillance systems are widely implemented. A backup system is an important part of your disaster-recovery plans. Basically, we need locks, safes, or security guards. Besides physical solutions, we also need to have electronic-security solutions. Here is a list of features to protect network security:

- ❑ Access control lists
- ❑ Authentication procedures
- ❑ Password systems
- ❑ File and database security control
- ❑ Virus detection and eradication software
- ❑ Digital certificates
- ❑ Encryption
- ❑ Transaction logs
- ❑ User profiles
- ❑ Call-back or call-tracking system
- ❑ Automatic logoff
- ❑ Firewall
- ❑ SSL: Security-oriented protocols

Credits

8.2a   Office icons: Copyright © Depositphotos/vectorikart.

Information Retrieval, Telemedicine, and Consumer Health Informatics

Information Retrieval

"Knowledge is of two kinds: we know a subject ourselves, or we know where we can find information upon it," said Samuel Johnson. Information retrieval has become more and more important for everyone now. The good news is that we have powerful information-retrieval tools, such as search engines. For example, we can easily search any topics from the Google website if we have internet access. Similar search engines are Bing from Microsoft, Yahoo search, Wikipedia, etc.

We can retrieve many kinds of information through search engines such as Google. There are different types of searches. For example, we want to find out the weather tomorrow, and we need to have only one relevant information source. In order to measure this type of search, we create a concept: precise rate, which is the retrieved documents that are also relevant divided by the number of retrieved documents. If we retrieve two websites, only one is relevant. The precise rate is 50 percent. For weather searches, we hope the search engines have a high precise rate. Another type of search may hope to find all related information. For example, a Ph.D. student wants to find all related research for his dissertation topic. He does not want to spend several years on one topic and find it out later that similar ideas were studied and published. The "recall" rate is retrieved documents that are also relevant divided by the number of relevant documents. If there are 100 relevant papers on a topic, and the search engine retrieved 60 papers, then the recall rate is 60 percent. After we have concepts such as recall rate or precise rate, we can compare the performance of search engines. For example, everyone can give a try to find out which is better between Google search and Bing search. It depends on the type of search questions.

In general, all citizens are consumers of health information to prevent diseases and promote health. Healthcare providers also have needs for information retrieval. There is a new clinical workflow, evidence-based medicine (EBM), which is used to integrate individual clinical expertise with the best available external clinical evidence from systematic research. In the EBM process, physicians phrase a clinical question that is relevant and answerable. Then they identify (retrieve) evidence (studies in articles) that address the question. Information technology (internet or search engines) can help individual physicians gain better access to evidence. Physicians will critically appraise the evidence to determine whether it applies to the patient.

Telemedicine

Telemedicine can reduce the distance between the patients and healthcare providers with informatics, and it could reduce travel costs. One application is to provide health information. For example, web-based information (knowledge) resources were developed, such as Medline. In addition, patients can remotely access their EMR, such as lab test results or medication renew. We also have social networks for chat groups or consumer-health networks. We can have personal clinical electronic communications with healthcare providers, such as emails or messages. Smartphones are widely used, and more and more health applications are being developed for smartphones. For example, appointments with physicians can be scheduled using smartphone technology.

One type of telemedicine application is remote monitoring. For example, we can use telemedicine techniques to achieve remote monitoring of pacemakers. For diabetes or asthma patients, many health devices can remotely monitor patients' medications and health status at home. More wearable technology has been developed recently. For example, smart watches can measure hypertension, patients' blood pressure, or heart rate anywhere and at any time and can send the information to healthcare providers remotely.

Remote interpretation is another area for telemedicine applications. For instance, physicians can remotely interpret radiographic studies and other images, such as dermatologic and retinal photographs. We have success-ful telemedicine applications in tele-radiology and tele-dermatology areas which have positive return on investment.

In psychiatry, videoconferencing is a successful telemedicine application to reduce travel, yet it also allows doctors to observe a patient's facial expressions and body language. Tele-psychiatry is a growing trend in mental health.

When more intelligent robotics are available, telepresence applications will grow quickly. For example, remote surgery may be possible. However, a potential bottleneck for remote surgery is the bandwidth of a network. A slow network connection will be a barrier for remote-surgery applications.

Challenges to Telemedicine

The first challenge for telemedicine is Internet issues. For example, tele-medicine demands a high level of network security for data transmitted along the Internet. It requires high quality and integrity of network devices and pathways. Another issue is to ensure that every citizen has access to the Internet. It may be a complex social or financial problem. Another challenge concerns licensure. U.S. medical licensure is state-based, while telemedicine crosses state boundaries. Finally, economics in telemedicine is a key challenge. Return on investment of telemedicine should be positive to maintain this trend. Normally, there is a high cost to initially set up the information system, and benefits in health are hard to measure. In addition, related reimbursement issues for telemedicine services in health insurance must be resolved.

Consumer Health Informatics

Consumer health informatics will become more important in the future as the trend in health care moves from treating patients' medical issues in a hospital setting to preventing medical problems at home or in the community. Consumers/citizens will be full partners in disease prevention, wellness promotion, and healthcare management. Healthcare providers will engage patient participation in health care and shared decision-making. Consumers will conduct self-help, such as self-monitoring, implementing therapy, or evaluating effects. In the future, consumers will have direct access to health information resources, such as EMR.

Consumer Informatics Applications

Specialized health-information websites are being developed to provide substantive and procedural knowledge about health problems and promising interventions, such as MEDLINE PLUS or WebMD. There are many consumer health networks which can connect with other people who share similar concerns and with their healthcare providers, such as networks for breast cancer patients (http://chess.chsra.wisc.edu/Chess/).

Challenges to Consumer Health

There are two major challenges for consumer health. The first one is the quality of health information and content credentialing in those websites. For the new industry, we need to have credentialing or certification to maintain the accuracy of health information. The related evaluation criteria are needed. Healthcare professionals can play a major role in consumer health issues, and they can serve as sources of content and provide guidance for patients. The second challenge is the imbalance of healthcare knowledge between healthcare providers and consumers. We need to improve health literacy for citizens. Hopefully, healthcare providers can become information brokers and interpreters for patients.

10

Project Management

What Is a Project?

A project is a cluster of related activities, and one of its typical features is the presence of a clear beginning and a clear ending in time. Means (money and personnel) are limited. The product that is to be delivered by the project will obtain its final description during the project. To manage a project, we have to deal with the people, process, problem, and product.

The key attributes of projects are time (on schedule), cost (on budget), and quality. To manage a project, first you should rank the key attributes. For example, to get a bachelor's degree is a project. One student ranks "time" as the first priority. Given fixed four years, he or she may choose an average GPA (quality) and adjust budget as necessary. Another student is a pre-medicine student and ranks "high GPA" as the first priority. Given the fixed high GPA (quality) requirement, he or she may spend four years and adjust budget (e.g., hire tutors) as necessary.

Software Project

Software development is a special project, which is to create a software system to deliver business value over a period of time. There are many components in software projects, such as the equipment (hardware), the computer programs (software), the data, and users of the system, and procedures to be applied by the users. Potentially, the software project can be complex. Quality requirement for software projects are high because the software actually will be used in the end, and it should be fully functional. Everything is changing continuously, and those changes may make software development harder. Normally, software is developed by a team. To manage a group project, you need to deal with communication issues among team members.

There are different levels of medical-software projects, as follows.
- ❑ On the personal level, that is, the physician, the nurse, and the patient
- ❑ The clinical department, the outpatient clinic, or the primary-care practice level
- ❑ The healthcare institution level (the hospital or an organization of healthcare providers)
- ❑ The regional level (country, state, or province)

People Issues in Projects

A software-project team has many people in it, such as project leader, information analysts, system and DB designers, system analysts, data architects, programmers, operators, etc. The level of talent on a project is often the strongest predictor of its results, and personnel shortfalls are one of the most severe project risks. We need to find the right people for the project. Who are the right people for a team? They should be open-minded, willing to learn, and dedicated to the project.

Difficulty of Projects

Sometimes it will be nice to know the difficulty of the project before you decide to participate in the project. The difficulty of a project depends on many things.
- ❑ Number of functions performed: small or large?
- ❑ Novelty of functions: standard or new approach?
- ❑ Number of users or concurrent accesses: small or large?
- ❑ Response time: off-line or real-time?

- ❏ Amount of data stored: small or large?
- ❏ Structure of data: simple or complex?
- ❏ Security: none or high?

Because of the complexity of application domain, many projects fail, due to scheduling issues, project cancellation, misunderstood business, or staff turnover. The project can go sour for many reasons, such as problematic communication. The team members may have different background knowledge or different vocabularies. They may not have completed user requirements or appropriated methodologies of development.

In order to avoid those failures in projects, we need to have a plan and systematically develop the project. We will introduce some project-management methodologies, such as software-engineering models, Microsoft Solution Framework (MSF), and Project Management Professional (PMP).

Waterfall Process Model [1]

In the software engineering, a waterfall process model (see Figure 10.1) has five stages: requirement, design, implementation, testing, and maintenance.

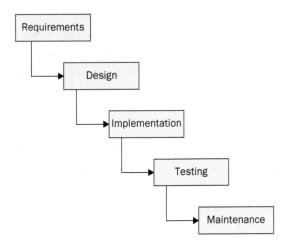

Figure 10.1 Waterfall Process in Software Engineering

Microsoft Solution Framework (MSF) [2]

The MSF Practitioner Exam (Certification) provides a framework that will assist organizations in successfully implementing technology solutions that meet or exceed the predefined vision and business objectives. There are five phases in this process model: envisioning, planning, developing, stabilizing, and deploying (see Figure 10.2).

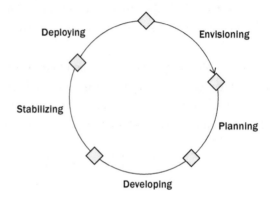

Figure 10.2 Microsoft Solution Framework (MSF) Process Model

At the end of the envisioning stage, a vision/scope needs to be approved. Vision is an unbounded view of what a solution may be. Scope identifies the parts of the vision that can be accomplished within the project constraints. When the first draft of a vision/scope document has been completed (including user interface mock-ups, etc.), it is circulated among the team, customer, and stakeholders for review.

At the end of the planning stage, a project plan will be approved. The team evaluates the products or technologies that will be used to build or deploy the solution. The functional specifications have been completed. A master project plan, which is a collection (or roll up) of plans from the various roles, has been completed.

In the developing stage, scope is completed, and the software has its first use. Executable source codes, installation scripts and configuration settings for deployment, frozen functional specification, and test specifications and test cases have been completed.

In the stabilizing and deploying stage, software is released. Golden release, release notes, performance-support elements, test results and testing tools, source code and executables, project documents, and milestone review have been completed.

MSF also provides some team models. Figure 10.3 illustrates how coordination occurs either with a business focus or a technology focus. It lists many units, such as product management, user education, testing, program management, development, and logistics management.

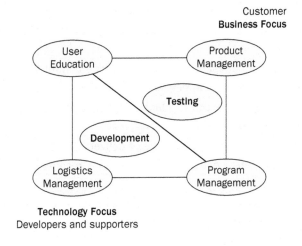

Figure 10.3 MSF Team Model

The MSF Risk Management model has six logical steps through which the team manages current risks, plans and executes risk management strategies, and captures knowledge for the enterprise. It need to firstly identify risks, analyze and prioritize them, plan and schedule the risk management strategies, track and report on them, control them, and finally learn from previous risk management.

Project Management Professional (PMP) [3]

The Project Management Professional Certification Exam (PMP) includes six units, as follows.

1. Project Initiation: Determine project goals, deliverables, process outputs, document constraints, and assumptions; define strategy; identify performance criteria; determine resource requirements; define budget; and produce formal documentation.
2. Project Planning: Refine project, develop resource-management plan, refine time and cost estimates, establish project controls, develop project plan, and obtain plan approval.
3. Project Execution: Commit resources, implement resources, manage progress, communicate progress, and implement quality assurance procedures.
4. Project Control: Measure performance, refine control limits, take corrective action, evaluate effectiveness of corrective action, ensure plan compliance, reassess control plans, respond to risk-event triggers, and monitor project activity.
5. Project Closing: Obtain acceptance of deliverables, document lessons learned, facilitate closure, preserve product records and tools, and release resources.
6. Project Responsibility: Ensure integrity, contribute to knowledge base, apply professional knowledge, balance stakeholder interests, and respect differences.

References

Benington, Herbert D. "Production of Large Computer Programs." *IEEE Annals of the History of Computing* (IEEE Educational Activities Department) 5 (4) (October 1, 1983): 350–361.

Turner, Michael S. V. *Microsoft Solutions Framework Essentials: Building Successful Technology Solutions*. Microsoft Press, 2006.

Project Management Professional (PMP) Examination Specification. Project Management Institute. September 2005.

11

Medical Software Projects and EMR Challenges

The application of medical informatics is to identify unmet medical needs and implement IT as a solution. The first step is to identify unmet medical needs. In hospitals, there are many clinical departments, such as nephrology, endocrinology, hematology, cardiology, dermatology, gastroenterology, respiratory, etc. There are also clinical supporting departments, such as pathology, function laboratories, radiology, and pharmacy. Specific tasks are encountered in each clinical department or clinical supporting department. The second step is to implement IT as a solution to meet the needs.

Some medical informatics applications include:

Diabetes

More than 29 million Americans, or nine percent of the population, has diabetes. The clinician enters the therapy plan, including time schedules for glucose measurements, a schema with dosages for insulin injection, dietary recommendations, and advice for physical exercise.

Information technology can assist diabetic patients at home by giving them therapeutic directions. Based on the plan, the computer system can remind patients at the appropriate time about certain actions that must be taken. The system can perform some automatic measurements and store the results and provide some overviews of patient activities or profiles.

Hemophilia

Hemophilia is a disorder in which a patient's blood doesn't clot normally because it lacks sufficient blood-clotting proteins. To treat hemophilia patients, we need to provide immediate overviews of the most recent bleeding events and related treatment information. It is immediately apparent which body sites require preventive action because of frequent bleeding.

A hemophilia-patient database will be very helpful. It should include data on site of bleeding and type and dosage of the administered drugs, etc. The information system should automatically produce reminders for patients to present themselves for regular checkups and produce reports for the national hemophilia register.

Neurology

Chronic daily headache (CDH) is a fairly common disorder. It results in significant pain and suffering with substantial impact on quality of life and enormous economic costs to society. The information system can support standardized recording of related factors, signs, and symptoms, which are essential for a better insight into the causes, influencing factors, and treatment of CDH.

Cosmetic Surgery

Before surgery, video images and X-rays of the patient are taken. The interactive program allows surgeons view the effects of various surgical procedures on the patient's body. The various possibilities are proposed and discussed. Once the choice has been made, the application provides details about the surgical procedures.

Intensive Care Unit (ICU)

ICU is a data-intensive environment with the need to monitor cardiovascular functions, respiratory functions, renal functions, brain functions, fluid balance, blood parameters, etc.

Computers can centralize the information in a comprehensive fashion. IT can help with data acquisition, error checking, and information display. It also can provide better insight and understand a large amount of information and get key data quickly. The information can remind the ICU team of treatment that need to be given at a certain time, based on protocols. The computer can share data for other purposes and be integrated with other systems.

Challenges of Implementing EMR

In the last chapter, we will discuss some challenges of implementing EMR. To integrate EMR into the busy clinical workflow, developers must thoroughly understand clinicians' information needs and workflows in the various health-care settings. We have to develop intuitive and efficient user interfaces to increase users' acceptance. In addition, we need consistent standards to reduce development costs, increase integration, and facilitate the collection of meaningful aggregate data. To implement EMR, major areas of concern in EMR are privacy and security. We should comply with HIPAA's privacy and security regulations. One of barriers is that the initial cost of EMR systems is high. It's difficult to determine the scalability and longevity of benefits in health care. There are risks in transitions. The good news is that U.S. many incentives are offered to provide reimbursement to healthcare providers who establish meaningful-use EMR systems. Healthcare providers need continuous support from software companies after they install their EMR systems. The transience of vendors of EMR is a major concern for business continuity in hospitals. Now it is a safe decision to purchase EMR products from large companies and not worry that a small company will go bankrupt. Healthcare providers need to know the key functions of EMR systems before they purchase these systems. In order to improve the quality of EMR in the long run, we need to have a way to provide systematic assessments of EMR. Unfortunately, we do not have many evaluation studies on the quality of EMR systems. People do not like changes, and physicians have shown some resistance to the use of EMR systems. For example, data entry may take extra time, and time is the most precious commodity to physicians. At the organizational level, the key challenges have been managing the complex applications and computer networks. Interpersonal challenges are much more daunting than managing the technology itself.

Appendix A: Homework

Homework 1:

Please briefly describe a personal computer (PC), which may be your computer at home or a PC in the computer labs at campus.

You should find out
- How fast the PC works
- How large storage systems are (memory, hard drive ...)
- And more ...

Homework 2:

Assume that you are planning to develop a laboratory database which will maintain the data that the lab generates, support the faculty and students who conduct experiments and research, and facilitate cooperation and sharing of information between labs.

Please identify the important things (objects) in a lab as completely as possible, such as, "equipment," "personnel," etc. Also, you should list attributes for those objects.

Homework 3:

A vehicle rental company wishes to create a database to monitor the renting of vehicles to clients. Each outlet has a stock of vehicles for rent that may be rented by clients for various periods of time from a minimum of four hours to a maximum of six months. Each rental agreement between a client and company is uniquely identified using a rental number. A client must take out insurance coverage for each vehicle rental period.

The entities are identified as the following:
- Outlet
- Vehicle
- Client
- Rental agreement
- Insurance

Please identify the relationships among the entities and draw an ER diagram for this vehicle rental company.

Homework 4:

Some transactions in an online bookstore are shown in a large table below. For example, a transaction shows that a customer bought a book titled *Red Word* for $52.00 and another book, *Rock Story,* for $83 on September 1, 2003. This customer's name is Robert, and his home address is "12 1st Street".

Trans#	Date	Name	Address	Quant1	book1name	Amt1	Quant2	Book2name	Amt2
1001	9/1/2003	Robert	12 1st St.	1	Red Word	52.00	2	Rock Story	83.00
1005	9/2/2003	Tanya	45 3rd St.	1	Jame's House	62.00	1	Blue Sky	45.00
1023	9/8/2003	Robert	3 2nd St.	2	Jaws	100.00			

Please normalize this table to the first, second, and third normal forms. All tables, including the data, in different stages (first, second, and third) should be provided during the normalization.

Homework 5:

The housing office of a university wishes to create a database to monitor the allocation of accommodations to students. Students may rent a room in a hall of residence. New lease agreements are negotiated with rental periods and rates. The students are sent an invoice at the start of each semester.

The entities are identified as following,
- Student
- Lease
- Room
- Hall
- Invoice

Please identify the relationships among the entities and draw an ER diagram for the housing office.

Homework 6:

What are reasons to have physicians enter orders directly into an EMR system?

Homework 7:

What are network security solutions? (Include both physical and software solutions.)

Homework 8:

Telemedicine is the use of information and communications technology to provide healthcare services to individuals who are some distance from the healthcare provider. Please use the Internet to find one telemedicine application and briefly describe it.

Homework 9:

Use the Internet and other online sources to find information about certifications of "Project Management" and briefly describe them.

Homework 10:

What are some of the challenges in implementing EMR?

Introduction to Healthcare Information Technology (First Edition)

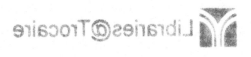

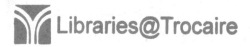

Libraries@Trocaire

CPSIA information can be obtained
at www.ICGtesting.com
Printed in the USA
LVOW05s1426090517
533872LV00006B/40/P